NO GYM? PROBLEM!

THE DIY FITNESS BIBLE

By the same author

Military Fitness
Live Long, Live Strong

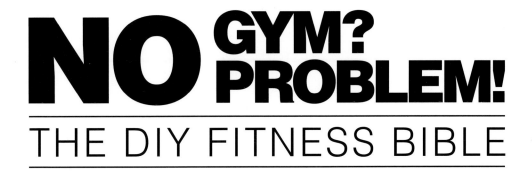

NO GYM? PROBLEM!

THE DIY FITNESS BIBLE

PATRICK DALE

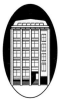

ROBERT HALE • LONDON

© Patrick Dale 2013
First published in Great Britain 2013

ISBN 978-0-7198-1070-1

Robert Hale Limited
Clerkenwell House
Clerkenwell Green
London EC1R 0HT

www.halebooks.com

A catalogue record for this book is available from the British Library

2 4 6 8 10 9 7 5 3 1

Typeset by Eurodesign
Printed in India by Imprint Digital Limited

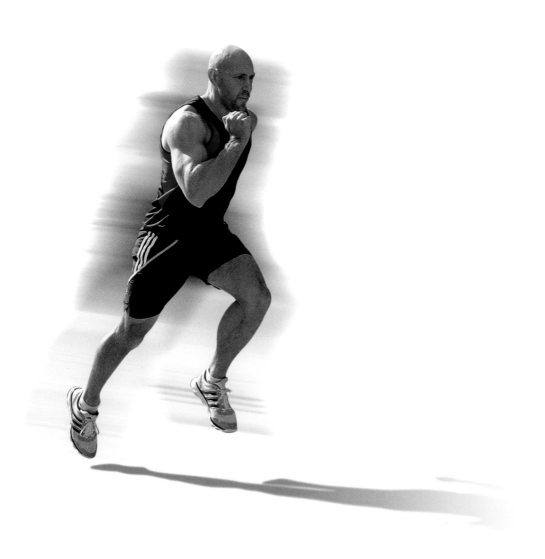

Contents

Do you have to join a gym to develop fitness and strength?

The modern fitness industry is in its infancy. As little as thirty years ago, the mega-gyms and fitness palaces that are now in virtually every city and town were unheard of. If you wanted a place to work out, you headed off to the local 'spit and sawdust' weightlifting or bodybuilding gym where you would most likely find little more than barbells, dumb-bells, benches and the ubiquitous wall bars. Public leisure centres weren't much better. I fondly remember, as a wet-behind-the-ears gym instructor, taking groups for inductions in the new and grandly named 'fitness suite' at my local leisure centre where an eight-station multi-gym had just been installed. Having only eight stations, exercisers had to book in advance to come in and work out – hardly convenient!

Fast forward to today and there are dozens if not hundreds of companies offering amazing fitness facilities. Competition is fierce and it's not uncommon to find numerous gyms in close proximity, all vying for your membership fees.

Despite sales pitches to the contrary, the majority of these gyms are very similar. They are built to a formula designed to excite and impress you. The highest paid members of staff are generally the sales team and it's their job, using proven sales techniques, to get you to sign on the dotted line and commit to a membership.

Just as supermarkets are designed in such a way that you are, for all intents and purposes, corralled around the aisles past every type of foodstuff and end up buying things you didn't even want, modern gyms are designed to focus your attention in a certain direction. Once you have passed the reception desk and strolled through the relaxing lounge and bar area, the chances are that the first thing you will see in a typical mega-gym is the cardio area. Spread out before you, like acres of chrome-coated giant hamster wheels, you'll see dozens of treadmills, exercise bikes, cross-trainers, stair-climbers, rowing machines and other state-of-the-art devices designed to increase your cardiovascular fitness and burn fat.

For many exercisers, this huge expanse of equipment will have them drooling and ready to sign on the dotted line right then and there. Most gym users believe that cardiovascular fitness (and therefore cardiovascular equipment) is the key to health and longevity and the gyms know this. That's why the cardio equipment is so prominent and abundant.

If that cornucopia of cardio kit hasn't convinced you to join the gym, you'll also find row upon row of selectorized strength-training equipment. Shiny, padded, smooth to use and designed to look as unthreatening as possible, there will be at least one machine for every muscle you will ever want to work and a whole lot more for muscles you didn't even know you had! Some gyms will offer multiple machines for each muscle group and even multiple ranges of machines from a variety of manufacturers.

And then, somewhere near the back of the gym and inevitably tucked away in the corner, you'll find the free-weights area. This is where the 'serious' exercisers hang out. For reasons that I've never fully understood, this area is often considered the reserve of male exercisers and those who consider themselves 'hardcore'. This is where the barbells and dumb-bells of old reside and this section can often appear to be a gym within a gym.

Modern gyms are jam-packed with equipment

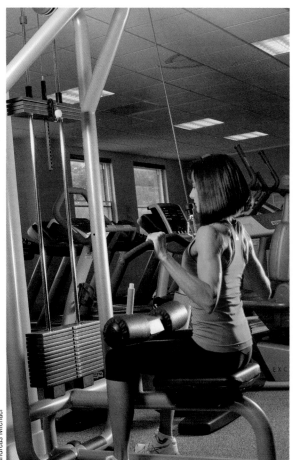

Andreas Michael

Frequenters of the free-weights area seldom venture out into the forest of chromed selectorized strength-training machines and those who have been seduced by the acres of beeping, flashing cardio equipment seldom cross over to where the 'real men' train - weird, but true. In much the same way that a vegan would probably not spend time at the butcher's counter at the supermarket, it's a case of never the twain shall meet!

Finally, on our tour of a typical modern gym, you'll come across the group exercise studio. This is where classes like body pump, aerobics, circuits and yoga take place. Chances are, if no class is currently happening, this room will be empty – a big, clear space just waiting to be used. Ironically, this area is probably the most versatile and useful place in the whole facility. In fact, if the rest of the equipment residing in the gym mysteriously disappeared overnight, so long as you had access to this space or one like it, you'd still be able to develop and maintain a high level of fitness.

No treadmill? Skipping (or jumping rope if you prefer) will keep your heart and lungs in

No Gym? No problem!

tip-top shape. Want to develop your upper body but don't have access to a bench and barbell/dumb-bells? The good old press-up will get the job done; no fuss, no bother. Legs need toning and strengthening? Look no further than the humble lunge or squat – no need to lose fitness simply because your favourite leg-press machine is unavailable.

The truth of the matter is you don't actually need any specialist equipment to develop and maintain a high level of fitness. The modern mega-gym is really only designed for one purpose – to relieve you of your money. It is, after all, the fitness industry, not the fitness charity! Modern exercise machines are simply designed to make exercise easier and more comfortable. And while there is nothing especially wrong with that, easier does not necessarily mean more effective.

Consider one of the most popular exercises seen in modern gyms today: the bench press. This exercise has only really been in existence since just after the Second World War but it has become a staple of virtually every man's training routine. The amount of weight you can bench press is a common topic of conversation amongst gym-goers.

The bench press is a chest exercise that also uses the shoulders and the triceps, located on the back of your upper arm. It involves lying on your back and lowering a weight from arm's length to your chest and then pressing it back to arm's length again. In terms of chest exercises, it is considered an important lift. However, if you consider the carryover of the bench press to the 'real world' you will see its actual value is somewhat overrated.

Firstly, consider the position in which the exercise is performed – supine or lying flat on your back. Unless you are training to take the place of a car jack, it's very unlikely this is a movement that you will ever be called upon to perform outside of the gym environment. It's not what experts call a functional exercise.

Secondly, how often do you actually push something away from you using only your arms and chest? In reality, pushing movements normally start all the way down at your feet, travel up through your midsection and it's only at the end of the movement that your chest, shoulders and arms get in on the action. Don't believe me? Try pushing a stalled car with just your arms!

Finally, let's talk safety. Bench pressing requires that you hold and support a potentially heavy weight over your chest. The weight has to be sufficiently heavy to be challenging. If, as often happens, you reach a level of fatigue that means you are no longer able to complete a repetition, you can find yourself in the unenviable position of having a heavy bar pressing down on your chest and no way to lift it off. At best this is embarrassing and at worse potentially life-threatening.

As a result, bench pressing is best performed with a spotter on hand. A spotter is someone who is prepared to stand over you and lend assistance if you run into difficulties. This means that the bench-press exercise becomes doubly labour intensive as you can't really train alone.

Let's compare the press-up to the bench press. Despite targeting the same muscles, the press-up also uses virtually every other muscle on the front of your body. From toes to nose, that's a whole lot of additional muscle power required. This means that, unlike the bench press, the press-up actually teaches you to push with your entire body – just like you would in nature. Then there is the fact that, during a press-up, your body moves through space rather than remaining stationary, as it does in the bench press. This type of movement places significant stress on your nervous system and, in exercise, nervous system stress is good. Movement through space will enhance your balance, coordination, intramuscular control, proprioception (the ability to sense where your limbs are without being able to see them) and your general athleticism.

Finally, consider the safety aspect of the press-up. If you work really hard and get to the point where you are unable to complete any further repetitions, all you need to do is bend your arms and lower your chest to the floor for a rest. No danger of being crushed. No requirement for a bodyguard-like spotter to lend a hand. You can safely perform press-ups on your own and pretty much anywhere you chose.

Don't misunderstand me – I'm no bench-press hater. In fact, I really like the exercise, and if you want to develop maximal strength in your upper-body pushing muscles then it's all but essential. However, for the vast majority of general exercisers and fitness enthusiasts, the press-up is actually a better choice as its benefits far outweigh those of the bench press. In exercise, I'm all about efficiency – and press-ups deliver more 'bang for your buck'.

People have exercised for literally thousands of years. Ancient Greek statues, Sanskrit texts and Roman mosaics all illustrate and describe how man has striven to better himself through regular physical exercise. However, it is only relatively recently that technological and scientific advancements have played a significant role in the pursuit of fitness and health.

It seems that, as with so many aspects of modern living, the more knowledge we gain regarding exercise, the more complicated that subject becomes. Type 'exercise' into your computer's search engine and you'll soon see what I mean. Exercise has been studied in remarkable depth and much of the information garnered has filtered through to the mainstream. Not so many years ago, this information was in the hands of a select number of coaches and experts and distributed on a 'need-to-know' basis. Now, in contrast, everyone has access to the same level of information and that's a real problem. Techniques, methods and exercises really only suitable for advanced or specialist exercisers are now readily available and are often practiced by people simply not ready for them. Exercise is, or should be, a healthy and life-affirming pursuit, but the wrong types of exercise, advanced training methods and certain exercise tools may, if used too early in an exerciser's career, result in frustration, disillusionment and even serious injury. It's often a case of too much or too advanced, too soon.

All of this information and all of the aforementioned grand facilities may lead you to conclude that the only way to get fit, strong and healthy is to join and train at a large and well-equipped gym. But is this actually true? Absolutely not. In reality, you don't need specialist equipment and you don't need a dedicated training area; you simply need your body and a small amount of space. You see, the truth of the matter is this: you are your own gym! And unlike a modern mega-gym, there are no membership fees, the doors are never closed, you get to train to whatever music you like and you don't have to queue to do your favourite exercise!

The ancient Romans didn't have access to scientifically designed exercise equipment, but they still managed to colonize much of the ancient world, marching and fighting their way across continents. As I detailed in my first book, *Military Fitness*, soldiers of old didn't do fancy exercises to hone and tone their bodies, they worked hard and smart instead.

In India, thousands of years ago, yogis were busy developing the first formalized form of exercise - yoga. Equipment use (straps, blocks, balls etc.) is a very recent development in yoga and in traditional forms all you use is a thin mat or towel for comfort. While yoga might not be all-encompassing in terms of physical benefits, it does prove that you really need very little in the way of equipment to achieve fitness and health.

Yoga – the original no-frills workout

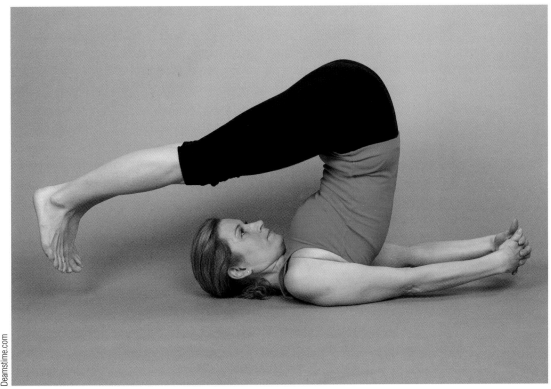

Deamstime.com

And it's not just the ancients who followed a very simple exercise routine that resulted in high levels of fitness. Modern military training is often very low-tech but still extremely effective. As a former Royal Marine, I seldom had access to well-equipped gyms. On deployment, we had little more than a few sandbags, rocks and whatever else we could scrounge from the local area. Did that mean that we had an excuse not to stay 'combat fit'? Did it heck!

There are many more examples of groups and individuals who have developed amazing levels of fitness and health using very little in the way of exercise equipment. Boxers, climbers, gymnasts, runners, martial artists and dancers have all achieved amazing levels of fitness and strength without setting foot in a mega-gym and you can do the same.

Gyms do offer some exercise advantages such as convenience, a wide range of exercise choices and an attractive socializing opportunity, but they can also distract you from doing what your body would actually benefit from most – effective exercise.

Effective exercise is often simple but does simple mean easy? Absolutely not. Simple exercises can be extremely challenging: burpees and handstand press-ups, for example. Anyone who tells you that you can achieve great results without paying your dues in sweat and effort is mistaken – or possibly lying! However, the simple application of effort can produce some amazing fitness benefits.

The aim of this book is to strip away the frippery and faff commonly associated with exercise and provide you with everything you need to get fit using an absolute minimum of exercise equipment – and in many cases none at all.

If you are looking for a book on the most advanced, complex and scientifically proven exercise methods around, I suggest that you put this book back on the bookshelf and choose something else instead. However, if you are looking for a guide to getting and staying fit at home, in your garage, in your garden or in your local park then you've made a great choice.

CHAPTER ONE

Pre-exercise considerations and precautions

Exercise is, by and large, a healthy and beneficial pursuit. By strengthening your heart, lungs and muscles you will improve not only your fitness but also your general physical well-being, which can lead to a reduced incidence of conditions such as high blood pressure, coronary heart disease, diabetes and obesity. However, exercise is not without risks. If you join a gym or employ the services of a personal trainer, you will probably be screened before you exercise to ensure any negative risks associated with exercise are minimized.

As you are likely to be exercising independently of any such supervision, it's important that you answer a few simple questions regarding your health and exercise history to ensure you are healthy enough to exercise. This questionnaire, called a Participation Activity Readiness Questionnaire or PAR-Q for short, will highlight any potential issues that may affect your ability to exercise safely.

If you answer yes to any of the following questions you should seek medical advice before starting this or any other exercise programme. A yes answer will not automatically preclude you from exercise. Chances are your doctor will say 'good for you – it's about time too, you lazy so-and-so!' and send you on your way. However, in some circumstances he/she may tell you that certain exercises are best avoided or that you should consider an easier, gentler form of exercise initially to improve your basic health and fitness. High blood pressure, for example, usually means that exercises that are isometric (or static) in nature or involve raising heavy loads above your head should be excluded from your workout as this type of movement can elevate your blood pressure further still.

Even if you 'pass' the PAR-Q with flying colours (not that it's THAT kind of test!), if you are new to exercise (or even if you are an old hand) it is essential that you listen to your body. Pay attention to how you feel on a day to day basis and make sure you not only listen but also act upon the messages your body is sending you.

If you experience any untoward aches and pains, feel light-headed during exercise, feel ill in any way, are suffering a respiratory infection or believe that your ability to exercise safely is compromised in any way, you should skip exercising that day and only start back when you are feeling a hundred per cent.

Exercising when unwell, for example, when you have a cold, can actually delay the recovery process and turn a seemingly minor ailment into something more serious. Colds and similar bugs put a strain on your heart and immune system. Exhaustive exercise while your body is already working harder than normal to rid itself of a germ, bug or virus is really not a good idea. You can't, contrary to popular belief, sweat out a cold. You can, however, prolong your suffering by not giving your body's immune system the time and resources it needs to make you well again.

There are no medals awarded for exercising when ill or injured so don't do it! Like any smart general knows, success on the battlefield is all about picking your battles and tactically withdrawing when you need to so you can come back stronger and better prepared to fight another day.

Please answer yes or no to the following questions…

1 Has your doctor ever said that you have a heart condition and that you should only do physical activity recommended by a doctor? Y/N

2 Do you feel pain in your chest when you do physical activity? Y/N

3 In the past month, have you had chest pain when you were not doing physical activity? Y/N

4 Do you lose your balance because of dizziness or do you ever lose consciousness? Y/N

5 Do you have a bone or joint problem (for example, back, knee or hip) that could be made worse by a change in your physical activity levels? Y/N

6 Is your doctor currently prescribing drugs (for example, water pills) for your blood pressure or heart condition? Y/N

7 Do you currently suffer or have you suffered in the past from high blood pressure? Y/N

8 Have you undergone any operations in the last twenty-four months? Y/N

9 Are you currently or have you recently been pregnant? Y/N

10 Are you currently taking any medication? Y/N

11 Have you had more than five consecutive days off work in the last twelve months? Y/N

No Gym? No problem!

12 Do you know of any other reason why you should not do physical activity? Y/N

13 Are you significantly (more than 30 lb/13.6 kg) overweight? Y/N

14 Have you been sedentary (inactive) for more than twenty-four consecutive months prior to starting this exercise programme? Y/N

15 Are you forty-five years of age or older and currently a non-exerciser? Y/N

If you have answered yes to any of the above questions, please provide details in the space below. A positive response does not automatically preclude you from exercise – it merely means that you should seek the okay from your doctor before starting an exercise routine.

CHAPTER TWO

The knowledge: Exercise principles, methods and training systems

In the introduction, I assured you that this isn't to be a book full of exercise science but, while that's true, if you are going to experience all the lauded benefits associated with exercise it is important that you adhere to the principles that underpin the science stuff I'm not going to talk about!

You see, even before sports science existed, fitness aficionados discovered that, to experience exercise success, you have to follow certain rules. We now know, because of sports science, what is going on inside your body during and as a result of exercise. This increase in scientific knowledge has subsequently proven that the old exercise principles are indeed valid.

However, just as you don't need to know how an internal combustion engine works to enjoy the benefits of driving a car, you don't need to know about sarcomere and sarcoplasmic hypertrophy (not made-up terms – this is real science!) to make your muscles stronger and to look more buff. Simply follow these principles safe in the knowledge that the science that underpins them is solid, well researched and thoroughly dull!

Overload

If you always do what you have always done, you'll always get what you always got. No, that isn't some philosophical Zen mind-bender but a truism relating to exercise and fitness. Without progressive overload there will be no long-term adaptation to the exercise you are performing or, in other words, unless you expose your body to ever-increasing degrees of exercise difficulty, you won't get any fitter. Subsequently, it could be argued that overload is the most important of the training variables.

If you do the same workout week after week and month after month, your body will only become as fit and strong as the workout you are performing demands. If you only ever do sets of ten press-ups or run a mile, that's exactly what your body will become fit for.

Failure to increase the amount or intensity of exercise you perform will result in hitting a plateau. You'll be stuck in a fitness rut and, as the somewhat melodramatic

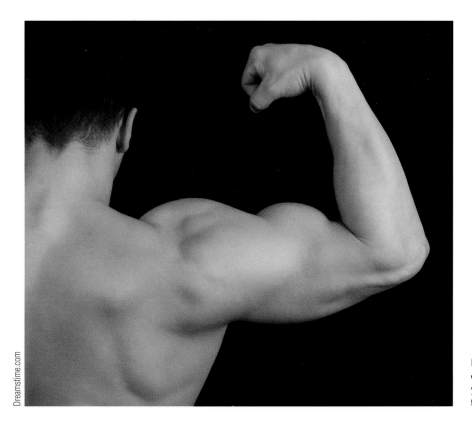

Dreamstime.com

If you want bigger or stronger muscles you must overload them!

saying goes, a rut is nothing more than a grave with the ends kicked out!

If you want to improve your fitness, you need to increase the difficulty of your workouts. This may mean running a little faster or further week by week, or striving to do more pull-ups. I'll provide you with plenty of examples of how to keep your fitness levels increasing steadily over the coming weeks and months but, remember, the key to fitness progress is doing a little more work than you are comfortable with. Only by 'pushing the envelope' will you experience continual fitness gains.

On this subject, I am frequently asked 'does exercise ever get any easier?' I normally get asked this at the water cooler or between sets of an exercise as I try to walk off the effects of hard training. Sadly, the answer is no. The perceived difficulty remains pretty much the same regardless of how fit you are. It's simply that your capacity for work increases as you get fitter. For a beginner, ten press-ups feels just as hard as fifty press-ups does for a more advanced exerciser. The only difference is that the more advanced person can do a higher volume of work before reaching the same degree of fatigue. So long as you are working hard by your own standards, your fitness will improve.

So how do you overload your body so that you get fitter? I'm glad you asked. The answer is to manipulate the characteristics of your workout – the so-called training variables.

Strength training exercise variables

- **Increase the intensity of exercise** – depending on the exercise, there are numerous ways to make a specific movement more challenging. You can use more weight, alter the position of your body, lengthen levers (i.e. move a weight further away from you or extend your base of support) or use a different exercise modality (i.e. switch from running to rowing).

- **Increase the volume of exercise** – if increasing the intensity of the exercise is not practical, keeping the intensity constant but doing more will provide an increase in overload. Adding a rep or two a week to your workouts or increasing the number of sets you perform will keep your muscles developing and improving

- **Increase the complexity of the exercise** – there are various versions of most exercises; from simple to very complex. Gradually progressing through these versions provides a logical and systematic way to make your workouts more demanding.

- **Change the target repetition range** – if, for example, you normally perform three sets of ten of a particular exercise, you will perform thirty reps in total. For variety and to stimulate progression, you could instead perform four sets of eight to total thirty-two repetitions, or two sets of fifteen. Either change will provide a sufficiently novel exercise stimulus and trigger fitness adaptations.

- **Reduce the recovery periods between sets** – in your initial workouts, you may find you need to take fairly lengthy rests between sets of each exercise. As you get fitter, you should start to use more structured rest intervals, for example, ninety seconds. Once you feel you are ready for a greater challenge, you can try resting less between sets. This means that you will start each subsequent set feeling slightly more fatigued, which will make your workout more demanding despite the fact you are not doing any more or any heavier exercises.

- **Increase workout frequency** – initially, you may find three workouts per week sufficiently challenging. However, after a few months of consistent exercise, and if your schedule allows, you could increase your workout frequency to four or even five workouts per week. Increasing workout frequency means you will be exposed to a higher weekly volume of exercise but ensure you still adhere to the principle of recovery and have at least one day a week off from training.

- **Decrease the speed of movement** – performing the same number of repetitions but at a slower speed will increase the length of time your muscles are under tension. For example, a set of ten squats where you take two seconds to descend and two seconds to ascend will take forty seconds to complete. If you slow down and take three seconds to lower and raise yourself, your set will take sixty seconds and as a result be more challenging.

- **Increase the speed of movement** – a strength exercise performed at speed often becomes a power exercise. Power exercises are inherently more demanding than slower strength exercises. For example, a squat performed at high speed becomes a squat jump and a fast press-up becomes a plyometric press-up. These are usually considered the most advanced versions of these particular exercises.

- **Reduce the base of support** – by moving your feet closer together or standing on one leg, you make standing exercises more demanding by increasing the balance requirement. This can make relatively light loads much more challenging. Also, progressing from two points of contact to a single point of contact will make exercises such as press-ups and squats very challenging indeed.
- **Introduce strength training systems** – training systems, detailed later in this chapter, are recognized methods designed to increase the intensity of your workouts. There are a variety of recognized training systems for you to try but be warned: they are really only suitable for advanced exercisers and, even then, they generally aren't suitable for day to day use. However, when you feel your workout needs to be kicked up a notch intensity-wise, the systems listed in this chapter will not disappoint.

Cardiovascular training variables

- **Increase the workout duration** – irrespective of the modality of exercise being performed, spending more time exercising will place greater demands on your heart, lungs and muscles. There is, however, a point of diminishing returns with cardiovascular exercise duration so, unless you are training to run a marathon, there is no reason to run marathon-like distances in training.
- **Increase speed** – rather than exercising for longer, you can exercise at a higher speed. This will drive your heart and breathing rate up and result in an increased level of aerobic fitness. Often, a short but hard cardiovascular workout can be at least as beneficial as a longer but more sedately paced one.
- **Increase workout frequency** – common exercise doctrine suggests that you should perform cardiovascular exercise three times a week. As you get fitter you may find it preferable to increase this to four or even five times per week. As with cardiovascular exercise duration, there is a point of diminishing returns with cardiovascular exercise frequency and three or four high-quality workouts can be at least as beneficial as five or six low-quality ones.
- **Change workout modality** – running is probably the most common cardiovascular exercise modality but there are plenty more to choose from. Swimming, cycling, skipping, circuit training and even rowing are all viable cardiovascular training options for the at-home exerciser. There is nothing wrong with running but, unless you are a running specialist, choosing alternative exercise modalities can only enhance your cardiovascular fitness.
- **Introduce cardiovascular training systems** – most cardiovascular exercise aficionados work at one speed – slow and steady. This type of training is often referred to as Long Slow Distance or LSD training and is not without merit but,

if you want to increase your fitness using LSD, you have little choice but to gradually increase the length of your workouts. As there is a limit to how much time you can realistically dedicate to exercise, it's worth considering other methods that will make your cardiovascular workouts more demanding. These methods include interval training, hill training, tempo running and Fartlek; all of which are discussed in Chapter 4 (see pages 77-83).

Back to the principles of exercise...

Specificity

For years, as a lecturer in personal training, I found it really hard to say the word 'specificity'. Even now I have to pause before using it in a lecture as it always seems to be waiting to trip me up! This is odd really because, as exercise principles go, specificity is actually one of the easiest to understand.

In simple terms, specificity means that you are fit for what you do. Your body responds to the stress you put on it and, make no mistake, exercise is a form of stress. The adaptations to exercise that you experience are dependent on the type of exercise you do. If you lift heavy objects that provide sufficient overload, your muscles will respond by becoming stronger. If you run, your ability to take in, transport and utilize oxygen improves and your cardiovascular fitness will improve. Stretch your muscles regularly and your flexibility will be enhanced.

For most exercisers, the *raison d'être* for exercise is to develop 'general fitness'. What constitutes general fitness? Here's a brief list:

- **Muscular strength** – the ability to generate force
- **Muscular power** – the ability to generate force at speed
- **Muscular endurance** – the ability to generate force for an extended period of time
- **Muscular flexibility** – the ability to take a joint or joints through a wide range of movement
- **Cardiovascular fitness** – the ability to take in, transport and use oxygen, also known as aerobic fitness
- **Coordination, agility, balance and proprioception** – selected functions of the nervous system which control quality of movement and collectively could be referred to as athleticism
- **Body composition** – not a true fitness component but one that many exercisers are interested in. Body composition is the relationship between the amount of fat and fat-free mass on your body. This is a much better indicator of health than scale weight which does not differentiate between fat, muscle, bone and water. Body composition is as much about diet as it is exercise and is addressed in Chapter 10

No Gym? No problem!

Some exercisers will make a point of exploiting the law of specificity to achieve a high level of one of the fitness components listed above. For example, a long distance runner may do little else but run and subsequently develop dizzyingly high levels of aerobic fitness. In contrast, a weightlifter might focus exclusively on developing strength.

While there is nothing especially wrong with specializing in this way, it could be argued that such a pursuit is not very healthy. The runner who has little in the way of strength or flexibility may well find that they are prone to injuries as a result of being, for all intents and purposes, weak. They may even find household chores like taking out the dustbin difficult as a result. Our weightlifter will have no such strength-related concerns but may find his heart and lungs feel like they are going to explode every time he has to walk anywhere or run for more than a few minutes.

Training in the style outlined in this book will not allow you to break any weightlifting records but you will get noticeably stronger. Likewise, you won't be winning marathons anytime soon but you will get fitter. I also doubt you'll be carrying off gold in gymnastics in the next Olympics but your agility and coordination will also improve. Holistic, all-encompassing training will not provide the peaks of development associated with specialist training but, if you want a good level of all-round fitness, to become a fitness decathlete if you will, you are in the right place!

Sleep – an important part of recovery

Recovery

Exercise is only part of the equation when working to improve your fitness. As discussed earlier, exercise is a stress that triggers your body to adapt so it is better able to cope with that stress when it experiences it again. In essence, getting fitter, be it strength, power or cardiovascular fitness, is a survival mechanism designed to make life easier for you – hence the importance of overload.

However, these adaptations do not occur while you exercise; they actually happen during the time between workouts and especially as you sleep. Exercise is merely the stimulus for change and those changes occur when your body is resting. That means that you should pay at least as much attention to your recovery as you do to your exercise.

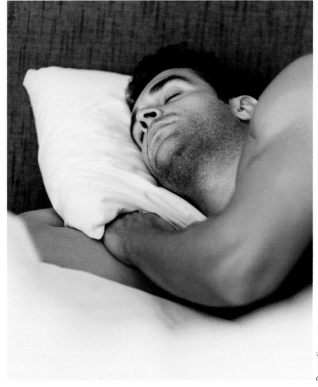

Dreamstime.com

As the saying goes, you can have too much of a good thing and that certainly holds true for exercise. As a naive and young triathlete, I pretty much derailed a promising competitive career by training too hard, too often and too long. If I felt that I wasn't making enough progress, I simply trained longer and harder.

In the end, the wheels fell off the wagon and I found myself completely incapable of even the lightest workout. I then had to take a long break from any form of strenuous physical activity. The thing is, I was always taking energy out of my body but never putting it back in.

Recovery is an essential ingredient in your pursuit of better fitness and health so don't neglect it. Follow these recovery rules to make sure you don't suffer the same physical crash that I did. Learn from my mistakes!

- **Don't be a slave to your schedule** - if you feel like you need to take an easy day or even an unscheduled day off from exercise then do it. Better to rest today and come back at full power tomorrow.
- **Eat a diet that is nutritionally dense** - fruits, vegetables and whole grains provide the essential nutrients required to ensure your body keeps running smoothly. If you are exercising hard, you need plenty of good nutrition to support your efforts. More on nutrition in Chapter 10.
- **Get enough sleep** - opinions vary as to how much sleep an adult requires but I wager that those who exercise hard need more than those who are mostly sedentary. Your body carries out the majority of its repair processes during your sleep. Anabolic (tissue repairing) hormone levels increase during sleep so too little sleep will narrow your window for post-exercise recovery. If you need to get more sleep, make an effort to go to bed earlier. An hour of sleep before midnight is worth two hours after, or so the saying goes.
- **Don't skip your cool-down** - cool-downs are discussed in Chapter 6 (see pages 132-138). The cool-down is the transition between exercising and returning your body to its pre-exercise state. Only when your body has returned to 'normal' can the process of recovery begin. Stopping your workout abruptly is not conducive to a full recovery so make sure you follow the cool-down guidelines described later in this book.
- **Consider your stress levels** - emotional stress affects your body in a similar way to the physical stress of exercise. The main difference is that exercise stress is usually in controlled and planned bouts interspersed with periods of recovery and stability whereas emotional stress can be never-ending. Adding emotional stress on top of physical stress is a sure-fire way to cause breakdown. I don't mean a mental breakdown or anything as severe, although that could be a possibility in some extreme cases. Rather, I mean that your ability to recover from exercise can become compromised if you are under continual, severe and unrelenting emotional stress. If you are suffering emotional stress due to work, family

or financial problems, you may need to moderate your exercise routine until you find ways of making that stress less impactful. Exercise can help alleviate low to moderate amounts of stress but more serious degrees of stress can be compounded by prolonged exercise.

Consistency

One swallow does not make a summer and, similarly, one workout or one week's worth of workouts won't do much for your fitness. Many beginner exercisers and a fair number of more experienced people make the mistake of going 'eyeballs out' for a few days or weeks but then fall off the exercise bandwagon. This is not the way to achieve lifelong fitness and health. The best workout in the world is nothing but wasted paper if you don't put it into practice – not just for a week or a month but for years on end.

One of the most important principles in exercise is that you cannot store fitness. The workout you performed yesterday, so long as it was sufficiently demanding to have provided the prerequisite overload, will trigger adaptations resulting in increased fitness. This process takes a couple of days and your new fitness level will peak around forty-eight to seventy-two hours after your workout. From this point onwards, if you fail to exercise again, there will be a slow but steady decline in fitness over the coming days and weeks until, after a couple of short months, you'll be back in the fitness doldrums and right where you started.

The only way to maintain your fitness is to keep up a consistent workout schedule. This is no quick fix but a lifelong undertaking. Your exercise choices, training methods and fitness goals may change over the years but it is a given that you need to 'keep on keeping on', otherwise you'll lose all those hard-won fitness gains.

So how do you maintain consistency? How do you avoid becoming an exercise dropout statistic? I'm glad you asked!

- **Choose activities you really enjoy** – don't like running? Try swimming. Not a fan of squats? Do lunges instead. Make sure whatever you choose to do is as enjoyable as possible. At the end of the day any exercise is better than no exercise so even if your choices are less than ideal, it's better to do something than nothing.
- **Set goals and targets** – exercise for exercise's sake is seldom effective. It's much better to exercise for a specific purpose. Setting goals is a highly personal matter but choosing and then working towards a goal can help keep you motivated. Examples of goals include training for and entering a local fun run or triathlon, exercising to reach your ideal weight or body composition, working to achieve a strength or muscular endurance standard (like the ability to perform fifty press-ups without stopping) or something as simple as clocking up five hours of

meaningful physical activity every week. What do you do when you reach your goals? Simply raise the bar and set some new ones!

- **Make an exercise appointment and don't break it** – my morning schedule goes something like this: get up at 6 a.m. and head out for a thirty-minute walk with my dogs. Get home and have a coffee and my vitamins while watching the day's news headlines. At 7.15 a.m., head outside to my 'gym', better known as my garage and driveway, and exercise for around forty-five minutes. At 8 a.m., have breakfast, grab a shower and be on my way to work for 9 a.m.. My 7.15 to 8.00 exercise appointment is all but set in stone. This is my time and I guard it jealously. I'd prefer a more leisurely start to my morning but I know that, if I move my workout to later in the day, something will inevitably come up and, before I know it, my planned workout will have to be postponed. For me, the key to my exercise consistency is making my workout a priority and getting it done before the rest of the day gets in the way. I'm not suggesting that this approach will suit everyone, especially if you aren't a morning person, but scheduling your exercise time really works.

- **Recruit a training partner** – misery loves company (!) so, instead of suffering alone, why not encourage a friend, work colleague or family member to exercise with you? If you follow the tip above and make an exercise commitment, not just to yourself but to your training partner, you are much more likely to keep it as you have just doubled your degree of accountability. A training partner can help you stick with your exercise schedule and also push you to work a little harder than you might do otherwise when training alone. This means you are much more likely to expose yourself to the all-important overload. Finally, a training partner can help share the financial burden of any exercise equipment you decide to buy. You won't need to buy much for this particular programme but, if nothing else, you'll have that option should you choose to make any purchases.

- **Start easy** – too many people make the mistake of letting their enthusiasm run away with them and dive headlong into a workout regime that is far too hard, too soon. Two marathon training sessions a day might sound like a really good idea when you are comfortably sat on your sofa planning next week's training but the reality is that such an advanced programme is probably going to be unsustainable and that means that your chances of maintaining consistency will take a nosedive. Instead, it's far better to start easy. Starting easy means that your initial workouts should be more about establishing a routine than having a major impact on your fitness. Remember, exercise is a lifelong undertaking so having a few easy weeks really isn't a big deal. It's better to walk before you run than run and fall flat on your face! Doing too much exercise, performing advanced exercises before you are ready or committing to working out too frequently can be real enthusiasm killers. Start slowly, build up gradually and take time to develop the exercise habit, otherwise it can be all over before you've even begun.

Periodization

Periodization simply means having a plan. In sports, athletes follow periodized plans so that they progress gradually towards their competitive goals. Each workout, each training week, each season and each year takes them closer to achieving their goals. If periodization works for athletes, it'll work for you.

In Chapter 9 there is a twelve-week progressive workout for you to follow. Each week builds on the preceding one so your fitness levels increase gradually but logically. What should you do when you reach the end of the twelve-week plan? Simply start over but increase the overall intensity of the plan. This is called linear periodization and is arguably the most effective way to ensure your fitness levels continue to increase month after month and year after year.

The alternative to periodization doesn't really have a name but I like to think of it as 'hit and hope' or 'speculative' exercise. The speculative exerciser heads off to train with little purpose or focus and does a bit of what they fancy on that particular day. Without any real rhyme or reason to their exercise selection, it's pretty much guaranteed that our hit and no-hoper will fail to adhere to any of the previously discussed exercise principles and subsequently they are unlikely to see much in the way of reward for their efforts.

Of course, that's not to say that, from time to time, it's not refreshing to exercise in a freeform way and do a little of what you fancy but, if this is how you train all the time, don't expect to see any meaningful progress. Just like having a map makes a journey easier and saves you getting lost and wasting time, having an exercise plan will ensure each and every workout you commit to doing takes you one step closer to your ultimate fitness goals.

By the end of this book you will have all the necessary tools required to create your own periodized plan. When in doubt, remember to start easy, build up gradually, change something about your workouts every three to four weeks and strive to work harder from one session to the next. If you do these simple things, you'll already be streets ahead of the vast majority of the 'hit and hope' workout brigade.

Part of developing a periodized training programme is knowing when and how to push hard and when to back off and coast. The occasional inclusion of recognized training systems, as detailed over the next few pages, is one such way to shake up your workouts.

Resistance training systems

Training systems are recognized set/rep/exercise combinations that are designed to increase the intensity of your workouts. Often associated with bodybuilders and other 'hardcore' exercisers, training systems can take your fitness to a new, higher level. But, be warned, training systems are TOUGH! Expect to feel sore for a few days after using a new training system. Some of the workouts in this book feature one or more of the following training systems whereas others are included so you can try them in your own workouts. Either way, training systems are a great tool for busting out of a rut and taking your training to a new, more intense, level!

System One – pyramids

Quite simply, pyramid training involves increasing the difficulty of an exercise and decreasing the reps performed set by set. Typically, pyramid training revolves around adjusting the weight you are using but this is not always the case and doesn't apply to bodyweight training where weight tends to be a constant value.

Pyramid training provides a great way to 'ease' into training as it basically involves a protracted warm-up that progresses into a demanding workout. This ensures you reach your toughest sets fully prepared for some hard work!

Example: ascending pyramid for muscular endurance using weights

- Set 1 – 20 reps with 15 kg
- Set 2 – 18 reps with 17.5 kg
- Set 3 – 15 reps with 20 kg
- Set 4 – 12 reps with 22.5 kg

After an ascending pyramid is performed, a descending pyramid could be completed where the trainee reduces the weights and increases the reps set by set.

Example: descending pyramid for muscular hypertrophy (bodybuilding) using weights

- Set 1 – 6 reps with 75 kg
- Set 2 – 8 reps with 70 kg
- Set 3 – 10 reps with 65 kg
- Set 4 – 12 reps with 60 kg

Example: bodyweight-only pyramid

- Set 1 – 20 press-ups on knees in box position
- Set 2 – 15 press-ups in ¾ press-up position
- Set 3 – 12 press-ups performed normally
- Set 4 – 10 press-ups with feet elevated
- Set 5 – 8 press-ups with clap

System Two – drop-sets

Drop-sets, also called strip-sets, is a method used to extend a set beyond its usual termination point. It takes advantage of the fact that, just because you can no longer lift a weight, it doesn't mean that your muscles are completely exhausted!

For example, if you were using 50 kg in the seated chest press and could just manage ten reps and not an eleventh, all that has happened is that you are no longer able to generate 50 kg of force. You could, however, probably generate 45 kg of force. Consequently, by reducing the working weight to 45 kg, you can continue the set beyond the point you normally would have stopped. After a few reps, 45 kg will cause your muscles to grind to a halt so you may reduce the weight to 40 kg and continue the set for a few more reps, thus pushing your muscles even further beyond the point by which they have normally given up the ghost.

To get the most out of drop-setting, it's important to try and reduce the resistance as quickly as possible once muscular failure has been reached. Machine exercises and dumb-bells are more useful than barbells as they allow the quick changing of weights, although with the use of a spotter or fixed-weight barbells it is possible to make drop-sets work with exercises such as bench presses and back squats. The amount you drop the weight by is intuitive and will come with practice but try to make sure that the drop isn't so great that your reps start to go up! It should take no more than five seconds to reduce the load for a given exercise, otherwise the muscles will recover too much and the effect will be lost.

Example: dumb-bell curls

- 10 reps (to failure) with 17.5 kg
- 1st drop – reduce weight to 15 kg
- 6 reps (to failure) with 15 kg
- 2nd drop – reduce weight to 12.5 kg
- 4 reps (to failure) with 12.5 kg
- 3rd drop – reduce weight to 10 kg
- 4 reps (to failure) with 10 kg

This constitutes a triple drop-set as the weight was reduced three times. It's worth noting that it's not necessary to perform this many drops – just reducing the weight once can be very effective.

Mechanical drop-sets

For bodyweight training, a useful variation of this training system is the mechanical drop-set. Instead of reducing the load between sets, the exercise is made easier to facilitate its continuation.

Examples:

- Feet elevated press-ups -> regular press-ups -> press-ups on knees -> press-ups against the wall
- Squat jumps -> regular squats -> wall 'ski' squats
- Jumping lunges -> lunges -> step-ups

- Overhand pull-ups -> underhand chin-ups -> body rows
- Swiss ball crunches -> crunches on the floor -> planks

With each of the examples above the loading (bodyweight) remains the same but the way the exercise is performed has changed so that the last example is the easiest version of the exercise.

Drop-sets are a great way to add intensity to a workout without having to use a spotter but, like all the other training systems, use them in moderation otherwise over-training and severe muscle soreness may result!

System Three – super-sets

Super-sets involve performing exercises back to back without any rest and can be used by anyone looking to add a new challenge to their workouts. Super-sets can be performed in a number of ways for a number of reasons...

Agonist super-sets

In this method, two exercises for the same muscle group are done back to back. As a general rule, the second exercise will be an easier/simpler exercise than the one that preceded it to allow for the residual fatigue that will be experienced. Examples of agonist super-sets include squat jumps followed by lunges, dips followed by press-ups or chin-ups followed by body rows. The second exercise increases the amount of work being done by the target muscle group and is effective for both muscular hypertrophy and increasing muscular endurance.

Antagonist super-sets

When using antagonist super-sets, opposing muscle groups are paired together. For example, press-ups may be paired with body rows or planks with sky divers. The benefit of this type of super-set is that the rest requirement is halved as the second exercise provides an active recovery from the preceding movement. This has the effect of allowing more work to be completed in the same time period or to make workouts shorter – both effects being beneficial to a wide variety of exercisers.

Non-competing super-sets

This method is a progression of the previous method. It pairs very dissimilar exercises together, e.g. chin-ups and crunches or press-ups and bicep curls. Again, the idea is to use the secondary exercise as an active recovery from the one that preceded it, thus making maximal use of the available time. This method is particularly well suited to strength training where sets are very short (one to five reps) and rest periods are very long (three to five minutes). By performing a second exercise during the lengthy rest periods, it's possible to make far better use of training time.

Lower-body/upper-body super-sets

This final super-set variation is very self-explanatory and is a useful tool for those looking to add a cardiovascular element to their resistance training or increase the calorific demands of their workout. Simply perform a lower-body exercise of your choice and immediately follow it with an upper-body exercise. Rest for thirty to sixty seconds before repeating. Always perform the lower-body exercise first as they tend to elevate the heart rate the most, making the method more effective.

System Four – Peripheral Heart Action training (PHA)

Looking for a do-it-all workout that strengthens muscles, improves fitness and burns a whole load of calories? Look no further than PHA training. PHA is a system of exercise which covers multiple fitness bases in one simple, albeit challenging, workout. When we exercise, oxygen-carrying blood is diverted to the working muscles preferentially. This 'shunting' of blood requires an increase in workload by the cardiovascular system (the heart and lungs). If, as in PHA training, we then immediately perform an exercise for a different muscle group, oxygenated blood has to be pumped to the new area of the body and the cardiovascular system again bears the brunt of the work. By strategically selecting muscle groups that are anatomically far apart (or peripheral) the heart and lungs have to work hard even though no actual cardiovascular exercise is being done.

Here is a template into which you can slot your favourite exercises. Note that the exercises should be what are known as 'compound', meaning that they utilize more than one joint and multiple muscle groups. The greater the number of joints and muscles involved, the more effective the workout.

- Any cardio for 5 minutes
- Leg exercise
- Upper-body pushing exercise
- Leg exercise
- Upper-body pulling exercise
- Any cardio for 5 minutes

Example: PHA workout 1

- Skip for 5 minutes
- Squats
- Press-ups
- Lunges
- Chin-ups
- Jog/skip for 5 minutes

Example: PHA workout 2

- Step-ups for 5 minutes
- Supine hip bridge
- Plyometric press-ups
- Squat jumps
- Body rows
- Jog/skip for 5 minutes

Each workout is a 'stand-alone' routine or the two could be combined into a single workout, although this is not for the faint-hearted!

When selecting repetition ranges, stick with moderate to high reps (twelve to twenty) as this will provide the greatest challenge to the cardiovascular system. Don't be surprised if the residual fatigue caused by the extra demands of PHA training requires that you reduce your working weights compared to when you perform the same exercises in a more traditional manner. Being out of breath can make even the simplest exercise more challenging!

To round off your PHA workout, feel free to add in any arm isolation or core work you feel is appropriate, but only after you have completed the main PHA segment. Remember though, although not trained directly, the muscles of the arms and the core have been exposed to a fair amount of work so their inclusion is not essential if time is an issue for you.

System Five – super slow

This method is an unusual one in that it requires a reduction in the weight and number of repetitions being performed to make an exercise more challenging. It sounds counter-intuitive but super slow is actually a very effective system, particularly when maximal weights or high repetitions are not suitable, e.g. with elderly exercisers or those suffering injuries.

The speed at which exercises are performed is correctly termed 'tempo' and the common tempo seen in most gyms is around 1:1, meaning that a weight is lifted in one second and then lowered in one second. Each rep (using a 1:1 tempo) would therefore take two seconds and a set of fifteen reps would take thirty seconds to complete.

Super-slow training requires a tempo of anywhere between 6:6 to 30:30 per rep! This very slow and deliberate tempo has a number of effects – momentum is all but eliminated from the performance of the exercise, tension is constantly applied to the target muscle and Time Under Tension (TUT) is increased significantly compared to traditional rep speeds. Slower tempos will initially require a reduction in weight used but don't let this fool you – super-slow workouts are still effective despite the low loads.

The super-slow chin and dip challenge – the two-minute upper-body workout!

If you can't do chins and dips, feel free to substitute with lat pull-downs and press-ups.

Chin-up - with an underhand, shoulder-width grip; start from a dead-hand with arms fully extended. Very slowly, begin to pull yourself up so that your chin rises up to and over the bar. Without any pause, slowly lower yourself back to the start position under control and without stopping moving at any time. Sounds easy enough doesn't it - just do one chin-up? The thing is, the rep is going to be performed using 30:30 tempo so that's thirty seconds up and then thirty seconds down again to total one minute.

Dip - using the same 30:30 tempo described above; start at the bottom position of the dip (or press-up) and slowly begin to extend your arms and press up into the top position. Without pausing at the top, begin to lower yourself back down into your original starting position.

If 30:30 tempo is too challenging for you at this point try 15:15 or 20:20 and gradually reduce your tempo by a second a workout until you can complete the challenge.

System Six – Escalating Density Training (EDT)

EDT is a training system that was developed by Charles Staley, a famous fitness trainer from America. According to Staley, the counting of sets, reps and rest intervals detracts from the main principle of exercise - overload. Staley's system of EDT eliminates these concepts and focuses on one factor - how much work is being done.

EDT requires the pairing of two dissimilar exercises and the use of a stopwatch. The exercises are performed in a loose back-to-back style for a pre-determined duration (called a Personal Record or PR zone). Rest periods are intuitive and the exercises are repeated as many times as possible in the allotted PR zone, e.g. fifteen minutes. At the end of the PR zone, the reps for each exercise are totted up and recorded. The next time this exercise session is performed, the idea is to complete more repetitions in the same time frame, using the same loads as before. The density of the workout has increased and therefore more overload has been achieved. When you can do twenty per cent more repetitions than your first attempt, it's time to increase the loading or select more demanding versions of your exercises.

When performing an EDT workout, it's important not to overstretch yourself in the first few minutes. Make sure that you keep a few reps in reserve as opposed to hitting muscular failure too soon. The idea is to do as many reps as possible in the allotted time and this is best done by resting as little as possible, so aim to do many sets of relatively low reps to achieve this. Staley suggests using a weight equal to your ten to twelve rep maximum but initially only performing six to eight reps per set. This allows multiple sets with minimal rest resulting in maximum workout density. As you near the end of the PR zone, start pushing the pace in an attempt to get as many reps as possible.

EDT is deceptively simple but the reality is a tough workout which requires focus and determination. It works very well for those seeking hypertrophy, muscle-building, muscular endurance or even strength if the correct loads are selected. One of the main benefits of EDT is that you know to the minute how long a workout is going to last so it's far easier to programme your exercise time.

By way of an example, here are a couple of EDT-style workouts...

Workout One
For the first fifteen-minute PR zone: dips and body rows
For the second fifteen-minute PR zone: squats and V sit-ups

Workout Two
For the first fifteen-minute PR zone: handstand press-ups and chin-ups
For the second fifteen-minute PR zone: lunges and hanging leg raises

EDT is a slightly unusual way of organizing your training but it is certainly effective, so give it a try – you might just like it!

System Seven – isometrics

An isometric contraction is where your muscles generate force but do not change in length. You are isometrically stronger than you are eccentrically (when your muscles lengthen) or concentrically (when your muscles shorten) which is, in this case, all but irrelevant as isometrics is also a valid and effective form of training!

Like isometric contractions, isometric exercise involves no movement. Your muscles generate tension, but the force is exerted against an immovable object or an equally strong opposing force - often an opposite limb, towel or wall.

To perform an isometric exercise, adopt the position you intend to use for the exercise and then contract your muscles as hard as possible against the opposing force. Do your best to generate as much tension as you can so that your muscles begin to fatigue within ten to thirty seconds. When you feel the force that you can generate begin to decline, push harder still for a final couple of seconds and then relax.

You might have seen people performing the wall squat, a very traditional and common isometric exercise and, coincidently, one of the most commonly misused. Most exercisers take a very leisurely approach to this exercise and all but lean on the wall while putting in very little effort. This is akin to doing bench presses with a bar that weighs one-tenth of your maximum - too easy! Instead, push as hard as you possibly can - try and shove your back through the wall! This will provide your muscles with more overload and more overload means improved fitness and strength.

The main advantage of isometric training is that you can do it almost anywhere as the exercises take very little space and, like most bodyweight exercises, little or no exercise equipment. Isometric exercises can be performed before or after regular bodyweight exercises, e.g. a set of squats followed by an isometric wall squat, to make a super-set, or performed as a stand-alone workout. Either way, isometric training is a great way to develop strength without the use of weights.

The main drawback of isometric training is that strength is only developed at around fifteen degrees above and below the angle at which the contraction occurs. For example, if you perform an isometric bicep curl by holding your elbow at ninety degrees, your strength will only improve through 75-105 degrees; a total of thirty degrees. To increase your strength through a broader range of movement, you will need to perform isometric holds at a variety of angles.

Another disadvantage of isometrics is that they tend to raise your blood pressure; something that is compounded if you mistakenly hold your breath at the same time. If you have high blood pressure then isometrics might not be for you and even if your blood pressure is normal, avoid holding your breath.

System Eight – ladders

A ladder is a very simple method of increasing the intensity of your workout gradually and safely and is especially applicable to bodyweight exercise. In ladder training, there are no weights to change or exercises to alternate between; you simply manipulate the number of reps you are going to perform in a very logical manner.

For example, this is a typical ladder workout for someone who is moderately good at pull-ups...

- Perform 1 pull-up - rest a few seconds
- Perform 2 pull-ups - rest a few seconds
- Perform 3 pull-ups - rest a few seconds
- Perform 4 pull-ups - rest a few seconds
- Perform 5 pull-ups - rest 2-3 minutes and then start again

You can apply ladder training to just about any exercise. For less demanding movements, you can increase the rep count accordingly...

- Perform 5 squats - rest a few seconds
- Perform 10 squats - rest a few seconds
- Perform 15 squats - rest a few seconds
- Perform 20 squats - rest a few seconds
- Perform 25 squats - rest 2-3 minutes and then start again

Adjust the number of rungs on your ladder according to your fitness level and always stop at the point where you know reaching the next rung is doubtful. So, using the above example, if twenty-five reps was feeling really tough, stop at that point. If, however, you felt that twenty five-reps left you still feeling reasonably comfortable, perform the next rung of thirty reps.

Descending ladders

Ladders can also be performed from the top down so your first set is the hardest and your final set the easiest.

Try this descending ladder workout, resting just long enough between sets that you can achieve the required number of reps in one attempt...

- 10 pull-ups
- 9 pull-ups
- 8 pull-ups
- 7 pull-ups
- 6 pull-ups
- 5 pull-ups
- 4 pull-ups
- 3 pull-ups
- 2 pull-ups
- 1 pull-up

System Nine – density blocks

Similar to the EDT (Escalating Density Training) system discussed above, density blocks pit your efforts against the clock so all you have to think about is cranking out more reps. The basic premise is that, after you have decided on an appropriate time frame or block, you simply perform as many good-quality reps as possible in that time. The next time you perform this workout, you should endeavour to complete a few more reps.

The duration of the time block is up to you, as is the number of blocks you perform per workout. Five to ten minutes are best but there is no reason why you cannot use shorter (or longer) blocks if appropriate.

Here are a couple of density block workouts to try...

The ten-minute burpee challenge

Perform as many burpees as possible in ten minutes. Rest when necessary but remember, that clock keeps ticking!

5BX (Five Basic Exercises) thirty-minute challenge

Perform as many reps as possible of the following exercises in five minutes. Rest one minute and then move on to the next exercise. Five exercises plus one minute rest between each equals thirty minutes.

1. Press-ups
2. Jumping lunges
3. V-sits
4. Body rows
5. Squat thrusts

System Ten – timed challenges

Timed challenges are a straight forward race to complete a predetermined number of reps in the fastest possible time. Similar to density blocks in that you set your own work/rest schedule, timed challenges are a great way to keep track of your fitness improvements as, if you complete the same number of reps in a faster time, you can be assured that you are getting fitter.

With any timed challenge, do your best to ensure that your exercise technique remains uniform from one workout to the next. If, for example, you performed your squats by descending to a thighs-parallel position one week and then only performed quarter-depth squats the next, you would probably perform more reps during the second workout as the exercise was easier and used a reduced range of movement. So, in a nutshell; NO CHEATING!

Here are a couple of timed challenges to try...

The hundred burpee challenge

Grind through the reps as fast as you can. Include/discard the press-up and/or jump as your fitness level dictates. Record your time on completion and try and beat it next time!

5/10/15/20 x 5 challenge

Perform five laps of the following circuit as fast as possible. Rest when necessary but remember the clock is ticking all the time...

- 5 burpees
- 10 pull-ups
- 15 squats
- 20 sit-ups

Record your time on completion and try and beat it next time.

So there you have it – ten methods you can use to spice up your workouts, push yourself to new levels of fitness or merely add something new to your regular workout routine. Remember, introduce these methods gradually and be conservative at first so as to avoid too much muscle soreness.

CHAPTER THREE

Low-tech/high-effect training tools ideal for home use

As I said at the outset, you are your own gym. Your body is an almost perfect exercise tool and, in many cases, is pretty much the only workout equipment you will ever need. That being said, sometimes it's nice to have a bit of variety available so you avoid boredom, have more exercise choice and can design a wider range of workouts.

Please do not think that any of the items detailed in this chapter are compulsory; they're not. They are simply things that have featured in my own training that have proved enjoyable to use and cost-effective, and they deliver results.

Sandbags can be shop-bought or made at home

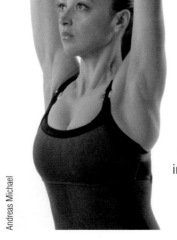

Sandbags

I used sandbags almost exclusively for a few months recently to field test them and see whether they really are a viable alternative to other, more traditional forms of weight-training equipment. I'm happy to report that, yes, they are!

You can make your own sandbags for next to nothing (instructions below) or alternatively buy one of the many commercial sandbags now available.

One of the things I especially liked about sandbag training was the way the sand shifts inside the bag as you exercise. This movement means you really have to 'lock down' your core and work hard to keep the load balanced. Subsequently, exercises such as overhead presses and squats become much more demanding and a light to moderate weight feels much heavier.

In addition, assuming you have a well-constructed sandbag, you can drop your weights with relative impunity as there are no hard edges to damage your floor. This makes sandbags ideal if you have to train indoors, in your lounge or spare room, for example.

Andreas Michael

Make your own sandbag

You'll need:

- An army/navy-type duffle bag (get one from an army surplus shop)
- A large bag of fine playground-quality sand
- A set of kitchen scales
- Twelve or more large, heavy-duty Ziploc-type bags (in multiples of three)
- A roll of duct tape

Take the duffle bag and cut all the handles off it. You want to grip the material rather than the handles so your hands get a workout along with the rest of your body.

Weigh out 5 kg/11 lb of sand and pour it into a Ziploc bag. Squeeze the air out of the bag and then seal it shut. Reinforce the zip with the duct tape. Try to ensure that the sand can still move around inside the bag and that you don't simply make sandbag blocks. This may mean that you have to put less sand in each bag if you only have access to smaller-sized Ziploc bags.

Place this bag inside another bag and seal the zip as before. Place this bag inside a third and final bag and tape the zip shut. This triple-bagging may seem excessive but take it from one who knows: sand in your eyes halfway through a set of overhead presses can really spoil your workout! Continue bagging up the rest of your sand until it is all safely triple-bagged. You now have your sand weights ready.

Feel free to make a variety of different-sized sand weights to make your sandbag truly adjustable. A couple of 10-kg bags, a couple of 5-kg and some 2-kg and 1-kg will mean you can fine tune the amount of weight according to the exercise you are performing and your current level of strength. Simply place as few or as many of the weights as you like in your duffle bag and tie shut using a belt, a piece of rope or something similar.

Adjustable fitness weights

I have used the term 'fitness weights' to differentiate between the Olympic bars and plates commonly found in commercial gyms and the smaller diameter bars and plates that are available from high-street sports shops. While these types of weights aren't really suitable for serious weightlifting, they are suitable for home use and are relatively cheap at around £1–2 per kilo.

As they are made of metal, these weights are long-lasting and can be used in conjunction with barbells or dumb-bells. While I don't suggest you need a full complement of weights for home use, 20–30 kg of plates and two dumb-bell handles with collars can add a reasonably priced extra dimension to your workouts.

As there is nothing that can really go wrong with metal bars and discs, there is no reason why you can't buy second-hand weights on eBay or from the classified ads in your local paper. It doesn't matter if they are rusty, dusty or chipped – as long as you have secure collars to hold the bars in place you have everything you need for a cheap but effective workout.

Kettlebells

Despite allusions to the contrary, kettlebells are not new. It's unclear exactly when someone decided it was a good idea to attach a handle to a cannonball but my research suggests that it was over 350 years ago and probably in Russia. This Russian origin is reinforced by the standard unit of measurement traditionally used when describing the weight of a kettlebell; the 'pood'. One pood equals 16.38 kg or 36.11 lb, no doubt the weight of a standard military cannonball at the time.

The Russians loved kettlebell lifting so much the Soviet Union even adopted it as a national sport, called *girya*, back in 1948. Other cultures also have a history of swinging and throwing heavy objects for exercise, including the Celts, Indians and English.

More recently, kettlebells have once again caught the imagination of exercisers and trainers around the world and are big news. Many well-known sports personalities are using them, as are some very in-shape actors and pop/rock stars.

Modern kettlebells are not really that different to the original Russian cannonballs from over 300 years ago. Essentially a weight with a handle, a kettlebell is like a dumb-bell, but the handle is above the weight instead of in between. Kettlebells are available in a variety of sizes from around 2 kg up to 40 kg or more. They are generally sold in fixed weights but some manufacturers have designed adjustable kettlebells to save you having to buy a lot of different 'bells.

Kettlebells are expensive, which made me think long and hard about including them in this list but, like the fitness weights described above, they are very hard-wearing and also extremely versatile. I don't think you need to go out and buy a range of kettlebells – unless you are thinking about using kettlebells exclusively. I own two kettlebells – a 16 kg and a 28 kg. I use the big one for squats, swings, carrying and pulling exercises and the lighter one for pressing and core exercises. I find that these two kettlebells give me enough exercise variation and choice to keep me interested without having to become a full-blown 'kettlebellophile'.

Suspension trainers

A suspension trainer is a device consisting of two straps that end in handles/foot loops that can be attached (or suspended) from a variety of anchor points such as a tree, a garage rafter or an eye-bolt fixed to a wall.

Once you have set up your suspension trainer, you can perform an enormous number of effective exercises for just about any part of your body.

Kettlebells – not necessarily cheap but very robust and versatile

Andreas Michael

Unlike weight training, where you use an external load to challenge your muscles, by adjusting your body position you use your own bodyweight as resistance (by shortening or lengthening the straps). If this sounds a lot like traditional bodyweight training that's because it is – but with a twist.

Because you are supporting your weight (via your feet or hands, depending on the exercise you are performing) on straps that are free to move in all directions, the stability demand of an exercise performed with a suspension trainer is much higher than the regular bodyweight exercise equivalent.

For example, when performing press-ups in the normal fashion, the floor is completely stable so all you have to do is concentrate on pushing with your arms and keeping your core braced. Press-ups using a suspension trainer are a much more challenging undertaking. In addition to lifting your bodyweight with your arms, chest and shoulders, you also have to contend with the handles constantly moving as you exercise. This places a lot of stress on the smaller and often overlooked stabilizers that lie in your shoulder joint – the rotator cuff. Every exercise performed using a suspension trainer will target your core and joint stabilizers, which can be beneficial for some exercisers.

Adjusting the difficulty of each exercise is as easy as shortening or lengthening the straps on your suspension trainer. The closer your centre of mass is to your base of support, the easier an exercise becomes. For example, in the press-up, by shortening the straps you bring your feet closer to the anchor point; you reduce the steepness of the angle of your torso and subsequently reduce the load on your arms. It's like moving from a regular floor press-up to a hands-on-the-wall press-up. Conversely, if you lengthen the lever arm by moving your feet and/or extending the straps, you can make exercises much more challenging. With practice, these adjustments can be achieved in mere seconds, which allows you to move quickly from one exercise to another.

Suspension trainers are light and portable, which makes them ideal for the exerciser on the move. However, some of the more recognizable models are expensive. There are, nevertheless, light commercial and home-use versions that are cheaper if less robust.

Big rocks

Although I would definitely refrain from using a big rock indoors, I see no reason why you couldn't use this most basic of exercise tools outdoors and for a great many exercises. I have a few big rocks in my garden that weigh between 15 and 25 kg (approximately – I've never weighed them) and I lift, carry, throw and press them like I would a sandbag or barbell.

Needless to say, dropping a big rock on your head is not recommended so I hesitate to recommend them for overhead presses, but the advantages of using a heavy

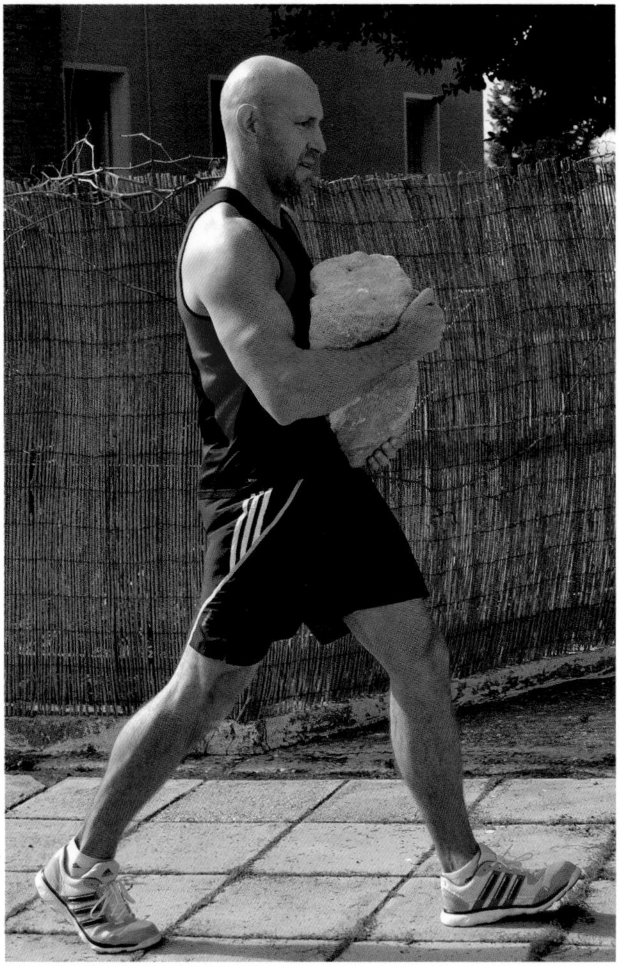

Victoria Cartwright

Big rocks are an unusual but effective workout tool

rock for strength training are plain to see – they're free and readily available.

As with all training, start light and progress slowly – never lift a rock if you have even the slightest doubt of being able to handle it safely. Dropping a rock, even on your toe, could cause a serious injury. If your rock is rough, consider wearing work gloves and an old training top that you don't mind snagging.

Tyres

Of all the tools in my no-frills workout arsenal, my favourite is my big, old tractor tyre. Ironically, this versatile and effective workout device was also the cheapest; in fact, it was FREE! Combined with a sledgehammer, a tyre provides a terrifically fun and stress-busting, lung-crushing, muscle-building workout without the need for deep pockets or having to go to the gym. What's not to like?

Tyres can usually be obtained free from your local tyre dealer. Just turn up and ask them for an old 4 x 4, SUV, tractor or truck tyre; the bigger the better. While the state of the tread is unimportant, make sure the sidewalls of your tyre are in good shape and are not damaged or degraded in any way.

If the tyre is too big to fit in your car you may have to pay a small delivery fee but, trust me, it's going to be worth it! The reason that old tyres can be obtained free of charge is that tyre dealers normally have to pay to have old tyres taken away so, in actuality, you are saving them money by relieving them of one.

Now you have your tyre safely installed in your garage, garden or on your drive (tyres are really only suitable for outdoor use) let's look at how you can make use of it...

Hitting a tyre with a sledgehammer is a fantastic total-body exercise. Use a light hammer (2-3 kg) to develop muscular endurance and cardiovascular fitness. Use a heavier hammer (5-7 kg) to develop strength and power.

Unless you have hands like sandpaper, you will also need a pair of work gloves for your tyre-hitting workouts but, other than the obvious tyre and hammer, you

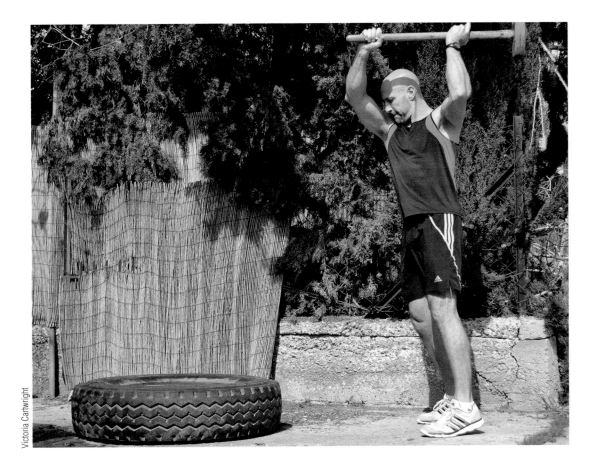

don't need anything else to develop a variety of fitness components.

Hitting a tyre with a hammer is easy to master; simply lay the tyre flat on the floor, grip the hammer firmly and swing it down hard against the wall of the tyre. The tyre will absorb the shock and make the hammer bounce back so you are quickly ready for another swing. Try to put your whole body behind the swing and remember to alternate which shoulder you swing the hammer from to ensure you develop both sides of your body. Your 'off' side will feel unnatural at first but persevere, otherwise you may end up with lopsided muscular development.

In addition to adding tyre strikes to a circuit by performing them in the usual sets and reps style, here are a few fun and effective hammer-and-tyre workout ideas for you to try...

- **Three-minute rounds** – using a light hammer, hit your tyre for three minutes and then rest for one. Repeat for three to five rounds. Swap shoulders periodically to save your grip and keep your body balanced.
- **Tabata intervals** – Tabata intervals are really quite simple but that doesn't mean easy! Hit the tyre as many times as you can in twenty seconds, rest for ten

Tyre and hammer workouts are great fun!

seconds and repeat for eight to ten sets. Don't let this short workout fool you -
it may just be the longest four or five minutes of your exercising life! Tabata intervals are explained in detail in Chapter 4 (see pages 81-82).

- **Timed challenges** - pick a timeframe, e.g. ten minutes, and see how many times
  you can hit the tyre in that time. Make a note of how many hits you manage and
  then try to beat that number when you repeat the workout.
- **Density challenges** - pick a number of hits, e.g. a hundred, and then try and
  execute those hits as quickly as possible. Make a note of how long it took you to
  complete your workout and try to beat that time when you repeat the workout.

As well as being a great way to hit stuff and not get into trouble (!) a tyre can be used
in other ways. You can flip it, jump in and out of it, jump over it, place your feet on
it for press-ups, stand inside it and lift it, carry it and drag it. If your tyre is relatively small you can even lift it above your head.

Fast feet are the key
to getting the most
from toe touches

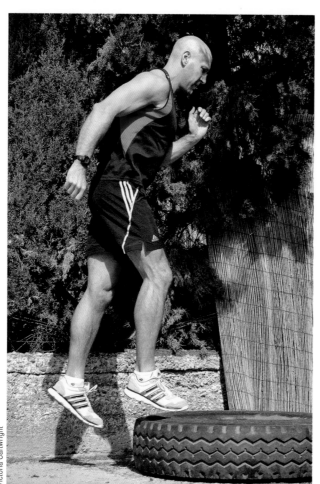

Victoria Cartwright

Here is a simple but effective workout
using nothing but a tyre and a hammer
that targets your entire body, will crank
your heart rate right up and also help you
burn a whole lot of calories...

Perform each exercise for thirty
seconds. Move rapidly between exercises
- no dilly-dallying! On completion of the
last exercise, rest for one minute and then
repeat. Perform three to five laps in total.
Feel free to adjust the work and rest
periods according to your level of fitness.

1. **Sledgehammer swings** - as described
   above.
2. **Toe touches** - stand next to your tyre
   with one foot resting on the sidewall.
   Jump lightly and switch legs so that,
   when you land, your foot position is
   reversed. Continue for the designated
   time.
3. **In and out jumps** - with your feet
   together, jump into the middle of your
   tyre and then out again to land on the
   opposite side. Quickly turn and repeat
   in the opposite direction.

No Gym? No problem!

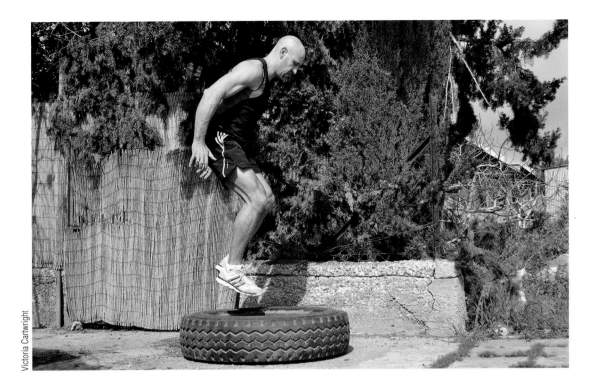

Victoria Cartwright

4. **Tyre flips** - with your feet hip-width apart, bend down and grab the underside of your tyre. Use your legs and arms to stand the tyre up and then forcefully push it over. Take a step forwards and repeat. If you are short on space, instead of flipping your tyre for distance, after each flip simply walk around it and flip it back again.

Tyre in and out jumps – great for your legs, heart and lungs

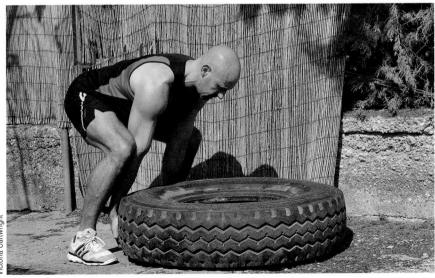

Victoria Cartwright

Tyre flips are great for total body conditioning

5. **Tyre deadlifts** – stand in the middle of your tyre and squat down. With your hands turned outwards, grasp the inside edge of the tyre. Keeping your arms straight, stand up. Push your hips back, bend your knees and put the tyre back down on the floor.

6. **Press-ups** – with your hands or feet resting on the tyre, perform press-ups in the normal fashion for the designated time. Press-ups with hands on the tyre are easier than press-ups with your feet on the tyre so choose the option that best matches your current fitness level.

A weighted vest will make even easy bodyweight exercises more challenging

As you can see, a tyre (especially when combined with a sledgehammer) is a powerful, versatile and effective exercise tool. If you have the space, one will make an excellent addition to your no-frills training armoury.

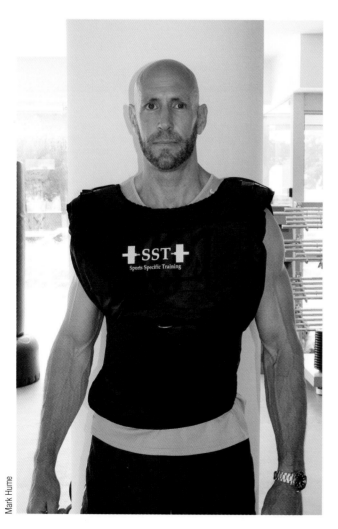

Mark Hume

Weighted vests

Bodyweight exercises are a great way to get in and stay in shape and in many cases provide sufficient overload to ensure your fitness levels soar. However, sometimes you may find that you get so good at an exercise that your bodyweight no longer provides sufficient overload and you don't want to have to perform very high rep sets. This is where a weighted vest comes in useful.

A weighted vest is normally made of tough nylon and has built-in pockets for metal ingots so you can make the vest lighter or heavier as required. They tend to be close fitting and use adjustable Velcro straps to keep them securely fitted to your body. Once you have your vest on, you should be able to move fairly normally and perform most bodyweight exercises in the usual way, the exception being prone exercises, such as back extensions, and supine exercises, such as crunches, as lying down in a weighted vest is not normally a comfortable experience!

Weighted vests come in all weights

No Gym? No problem!

and sizes but, as they are generally adjustable, it's worth buying the heaviest vest you can afford rather than a cheap, lightweight one that you will 'outgrow' in a few short months. My vest, the one pictured, has a 20-kg capacity and can be adjusted in 1-kg increments by simply sliding ingots in or out of the pockets. While it wasn't especially cheap, it does add a whole new level of intensity to bodyweight exercises like press-ups and squats and I have also used it when performing the tyre circuit detailed on pages 42–4.

If you prefer a low-cost alternative to a weighted vest, why not simply put some heavy books or even sandbag weights (as described on pages 36–7) in a backpack? It won't be as close-fitting or as comfortable as a well-designed weighted vest but it would still provide additional overload for many bodyweight exercises.

Skipping ropes

What do schoolgirls and some of the hardest men on the planet have in common? The surprising answer is skipping! Whether you are in a typical playground or a Mixed Martial Arts (MMA) gym, you'll see people skipping, or jumping rope if you want a slightly more manly term. So why the popularity of this low-tech form of exercise? The answer is simple – it works!

Skipping develops your cardiovascular conditioning, your eye-hand-foot coordination, strengthens your ankles, legs and shoulders and also burns a whole lot of calories. You can jump rope for extended periods to improve your aerobic fitness or for short, fast bursts to improve your anaerobic fitness. Tricks like double-unders and triple-unders (two or three turns of the rope per jump) will improve your leg power, and drills like high-knee sprints (where you lift your knees as you run) will improve your leg speed.

In addition to being a highly effective form of exercise, jumping rope is also very accessible and can be performed just about anywhere there is space to turn a rope. Skipping ropes are cheap – my favoured style of skipping rope costs less than £10 – and they seldom break. Once you have a good rope, you have a training partner that will last for years! Although learning to skip well can take a while, once mastered it is a skill that you never really forget.

One of the most important factors in skipping-rope training is making sure your rope is the right length for you. The wrong length rope can make your workout a frustrating start again/stop again affair so it pays to get your rope length right from the outset.

Stand on the middle of your rope with your feet together and your legs straight. Pull the handles up towards your armpits. If the ends of the handles touch your armpits, the rope is the right length for you. If it doesn't reach this level, the rope is too short and you should select another. If it is too long, tie a knot in the middle of the rope and check again. Tie as many knots as you need to make the rope the right

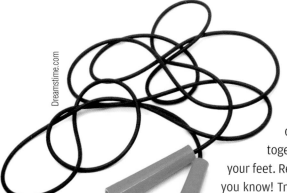

Skipping ropes – a
cheap and portable
exercise tool

length. Once you have your rope the right length, you are ready
to get started.

The most common technique fault I see with novice skip-
pers is a tendency to jump too high. The higher you jump, the
harder it is to time your rope turns. Ideally you should only just
clear the rope. Start with the rope behind you and your feet
together. Swing the rope overhead and jump over it as it approaches
your feet. Remember to just clear it – you aren't in a high-jump competition,
you know! Try to stick to one jump per rope turn and avoid the temptation
to 'double bounce' between revolutions. This will simply make it harder to
establish a smooth rope rhythm. Keep your hands down at hip-height and only
slightly away from your body. If you raise your hands much higher than this you
effectively shorten the rope and increase your likelihood of tripping.

As you become more proficient, try to increase the speed of your rope turns.
Once you can keep going for more than a few minutes you are ready to move onto
heel-toe action skipping – sometimes called the boxer's skip.

To make like Rocky and skip like a pro, start with your basic two-footed skipping
and then, when you are ready, kick one foot forwards so that you land with one heel
on the floor. Change legs on the next jump and continue alternating your feet in this
way for the duration of your workout. Once mastered, you'll be able to move
forwards, sideways, and backwards using this heel-toe action and it will act as a
linking move between other, more challenging, skipping drills.

There is a cornucopia of skipping tricks and drills to try but here are some of the
more commonly performed techniques that can be used to spice up your skipping-
rope training.

- **Knee-lift sprints** – these are a great drill for driving up your heart rate and
  making your rope workouts more demanding. From the basic heel-toe technique,
  transition into jogging on the spot. Lift your knees up in front of you so that your
  thighs are parallel to the floor. Pick up the pace and try to turn the rope as fast
  as possible while moving your feet as quickly as you can. Do not lean back when
  performing this drill. In fact, you may find you can skip faster if you lean forwards
  slightly.
- **Cross-overs** – jumping rope can make your shoulders ache, especially if you are
  new to this form of exercise or are skipping for long periods of time. Periodically
  crossing your arms can help to alleviate this discomfort. Stick with double-footed
  jumps when first trying this technique and then progress onto heel-toe when
  you feel ready. As you turn the rope and it passes overhead, cross your hands and
  form a loop. Jump through the loop and then uncross your hands. Because the
  loop in the rope is comparatively small, you may need to hunch your shoulders
  and tuck up slightly as you jump through it. Start off by performing single cross-

overs and then try to link multiple cross-overs together.

- **Double-unders** – a cool trick that can really crank up your heart rate and also develop lower-body jumping power, the double-under is a great way to make your skipping-rope training much more intense. Skip normally and, when you are ready, speed up the turn-rate of your rope and jump a little bit higher. You are aiming to turn the rope twice before landing. Initially, after a successful double-under, return to your normal skipping technique and then, when you are ready, perform another one. Once you have mastered single double-unders, try and link a few together. With practice, you will be able to do twenty or more in a row, which will have your your heart racing!

Once you are comfortable with each of these techniques, try mixing them into a freeform routine.

These are just a few of my favourite skipping-rope workouts…

- **Three-minute rounds** – inspired by the length of a typical round of boxing, skip for three minutes and then rest for one. Repeat for as many rounds as required.
- **Skipping and burpee descending pyramid** – this short but sweet workout is against the clock and really challenges your skipping ability and fitness. Perform ten burpees and then skip until you have performed fifty rope turns. Then do nine burpees followed by another fifty rope turns. Keep reducing the burpees by one until you reach one. This is a great 'finisher' at the end of a strength-training workout.
- **Jump and swing** – combining kettlebell swings and skipping, this no-frills workout is really effective but very simple. Set your timer so it bleeps every three minutes. Perform twenty to thirty kettlebell swings and then grab your rope and skip until the timer bleeps again. Perform another set of swings and repeat. Feel free to adjust the timings to suit your individual fitness level - two minutes works equally well and is more demanding as the skipping is actually the recovery part of this workout!
- **Skipping, press-ups and squats** – this workout is a great way to get a full-body training session into a very short time using nothing but a skipping rope and some clear floor space. Perform a continuous cycle of thirty seconds skipping/thirty seconds press-ups/thirty seconds skipping/thirty seconds squats. Continue for as long as you like. Ten cycles totals twenty minutes, making this a great 'in a hurry' workout.
- **Tabata skipping intervals** – my final favourite skipping-rope workout is the shortest but in many ways the hardest. Skip as fast as possible for twenty seconds (knee-lift sprints or double-unders are best) and then rest for ten seconds. Repeat for eight sets. If you aren't thoroughly exhausted at the end of this short but sharp workout, you weren't skipping fast enough!

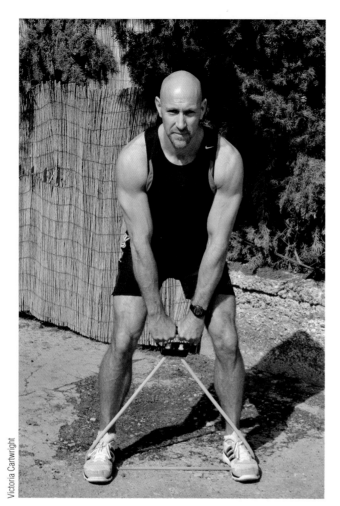

Resistance bands

Resistance bands can provide a veritable gym in a bag. Portable, cheap and readily available, you can use resistance bands in place of barbells and dumb-bells to perform many traditional weight-training exercises and also use them to replicate some resistance-machine exercises. All you need is some space and suitable anchor points.

Resistance bands come in two main varieties: closed loops and lengths with handles at each end. Both types are fairly interchangeable although the ones with handles can be used to replicate dumb-bell and barbell exercises more easily.

Available in a variety of strengths and lengths, you may need to shop around to find the best bands for your purposes but, once you have your bands, they last quite a long time and so represent a good investment. Many band sets come with door anchors, which make these versatile tools even more useful. By fixing your band at waist-height, you can perform exercises such as chest presses and rows, whereas a band set above head-height can be used to replicate lat pull-downs.

Resistance bands are a good alternative to more cumbersome free-weights

Exercises performed with bands feel slightly different to the same movement performed with free-weights. This is because, in most cases, free-weight exercises become easier as you near the end of a given repetition whereas band exercises are the opposite. This easy start/difficult finish means that bands are often prescribed as rehab devices for those suffering joint or muscle injuries. By and large they tend to be easier on your joints than more traditional forms of resistance training, useful if you are, like me, feeling a bit beaten up after years of hard training and/or sport.

Stability balls

You've probably seen these big inflatable balls at the gym or in sports shops and wondered whether they are actually anything more than an overgrown kid's toy. Interestingly, the first stability balls were actually made by an Italian toy-maker but that's really the end of the connection between stability balls and children's play-things. A stability ball can be used in so many different ways they really warrant a book all of their own but, suffice to say, they are very versatile.

The main reason stability balls are so effective is their inherent instability, as the name suggests. Exercising on an unstable surface means that you have to work much harder to keep yourself in balance. This means that small muscles, called stabilizers, which often go unused, must work overtime.

Press-ups and abdominal crunches are considerably more difficult when performed using a stability ball and there are a large number of specific stability-ball exercises as well. A stability ball can also be used as a replacement for a weight-training bench and is in many ways superior to this gym standard. Using a ball as a bench means you must push with both arms equally, use your core muscles to prevent unwanted movement and also means that your shoulder girdle (comprising your scapulae and clavicles) are free to move back and forth naturally whereas a bench pins them in place.

When stability balls first hit the fitness industry, they were embraced to such a degree that trainers not using them for every exercise under the sun were branded backwards. However, as is often the way with new fads, the initial enthusiasm for all things big and round soon wore off and now stability balls are much less popular. That's a shame because, while they might not be the be all and end all of exercise tools as many trainers initially believed, they are a cheap and effective workout device that would make a valuable addition to most home gyms.

Bag work – a great stress-buster!

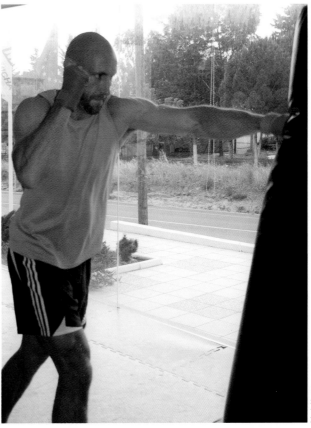

Mark Hume

Punchbags

Punching and kicking are very visceral activities, effective forms of exercise and great stress-busters. A few minutes of 'bag work' will soon have you puffing and panting. Punchbags can be hung from brackets bolted to a wall or from a tree in your garden; some are completely free-standing. It is also possible to make your own – see page 51.

Before you lay a hand on your punchbag, it's important you learn how to make a fist. Firstly, all of your punching force should be concentrated across the first two knuckles. Your other knuckles will come into contact with the bag but these two should bear the brunt of the force. Next, make sure you keep your wrists straight. Hitting with a bent wrist is a sure fire way to hurt yourself. Finally, never EVER hold your thumb inside your fingers when you make a fist. That's really going to hurt!

Hitting a punchbag means your hands are going to take some punishment. If you value the health of your carpals, metacarpals and phalanges, you should always wear bag gloves or, at the very least, wrap your hands in boxing hand-wraps. There are some very good and relatively cheap open-palmed MMA-style bag gloves around that leave your hands free so you can quickly transition from one exercise to another. If you are going to include bag work as part of a circuit, this type of glove is a good choice. If, however, you are going to just 'bang away' at your punchbag, regular closed-palm bag gloves will suffice.

Now, you COULD simply go bonkers and wail on your punchbag like it stole your car but, while that might be very satisfying, it won't be particularly productive as a form of exercise. You will get better results from using a more structured approach to your bag work...

- **Three-minute rounds** – throw combinations of various punches at various speeds for three minutes and then rest for one minute. Repeat for as many rounds as required. Add kicks, elbow and knee strikes if you know how.
- **Tabata bag work** – twenty seconds of rapid-fire punching followed by ten seconds of recovery. Repeat eight to ten times for a short but sweet workout. Just be glad the bag isn't fighting back!
- **Punching ladder** – throw one punch, pause, throw two punches and pause again. Continue adding a punch until you reach ten. Then work your way back down to one in the same fashion.
- **Density punching** – see how many blows you can land on your punchbag in a pre-determined time, e.g. sixty seconds. Rest a moment and then repeat. Try to achieve a similar number of strikes per round.
- **Punching burpee pyramid** – perform one burpee, throw two punches, perform two burpees, throw four punches, perform three burpees, throw six punches. Continue adding a burpee and performing double that amount of punches until you reach ten and twenty respectively. Do this against the clock, record your time and try to beat it when you repeat this workout.

Make your own punchbag

You'll need:

- An army/navy duffle bag
- Some carpet liner/underlay/old gym mat
- A craft knife
- Old clothes/rags
- Sand/gravel (optional)
- Rope
- Duct tape

Open the duffle bag and turn it inside out. Inspect all the seams to ensure the stitching is sound. Repair or reinforce any suspect stitching. Turn the bag the right side out.

Cut the carpet liner/underlay into strips that are as wide as the bag is long. Place the strips inside the bag so that it is fully lined. All the layers should overlap. Stand the duffle bag upright. If you use an old exercise mat, roll it into a loose tube and place it vertically in your duffle bag.

Stuff the old clothes/rags into the duffle bag. Make sure all the stuffing is inside the liner. Periodically put your foot into the bag and stomp down on the clothes to ensure that they are packed as tightly as possible. Continue stuffing and stomping them down until the bag is full.

If you want a heavier bag, add sand/gravel as you add the clothes/rags.

Tie off the top of the bag using the rope - use the middle of the rope so you can use the ends to tie your bag to an overhead beam or other suitable hanging place. Make sure the top of the bag is securely fastened. Wrap the duct tape around the bag. Start at one end and overlap each turn. Keep the duct tape tight and try to avoid any creases. Once the bag is covered you can place additional layers of tape over the most likely striking areas. Use the ropes to hang the punchbag from an appropriate anchor point. Make sure the anchor point is strong enough to support the weight of the bag.

Medicine balls

Available in a variety of weights, sizes and materials, medicine balls are a useful addition to your exercise armoury. They can be lifted, thrown and slammed to provide a great workout. As medicine balls are made from a variety of materials, it's worth knowing a little about each so you know what each one is most appropriate and, more importantly, if it is suited to you!

- **Leather** – while decidedly old fashioned, leather medicine balls are still available. They are tactile, they don't bounce and they are comfortable to use. However, while the no-bounce feature is useful if you are doing lots of throwing and catching exercises, they aren't weather-proof and can rot if allowed to become damp. A good choice for purists, but if you intend to exercise outside, a leather ball might not be the best choice.
- **Gel-filled** – gel-filled balls are generally cheap, soft and easy to handle. Their softness means they are excellent for using indoors and for throwing and catching exercises but they do not withstand heavy slamming exercises and are prone to splitting. If you intend to treat your medicine ball roughly, a gel-filled one won't last very long and may even leave a mess on your floor.
- **Rubber** – firm, strong and thick, rubber medicine balls are hard-wearing. I have one that has seen some pretty extreme use and, despite being ten years old, it's still going strong. Rubber medicine balls are firm and moderately bouncy, which makes them ideal for slamming-type exercises, but because they are so solid, some users find that they cause sore hands when caught at speed.
- **With handles** – some medicine balls, particularly moulded rubber ones, have built-in handles. This means you can lift and swing them like kettlebells, making them seemingly very versatile. On the downside, these handles mean the ball won't bounce uniformly and the uneven surface makes it difficult, if not dangerous, to catch. If you want a medicine ball that you intend to use as a kettle-bell or dumb-bell then these handled balls are fine, but if you want a medicine ball to throw, slam and catch don't buy one of these.
- **Tornado balls** – a relatively new development, a tornado ball is a medicine ball with a cord handle threaded through its centre – imagine a large, round, soap on a rope! Tornado balls can be used like regular medicine balls but can also be swung like a rope-handled hammer. They are designed to improve rotational strength and are very good for this purpose although you can experience similar benefits by putting your regular medicine ball in a strong bag or using a sledge-hammer.

Make your own medicine ball
You'll need:

- A basketball
- Sand or gravel
- Rubber cement
- A sharp knife
- Duct tape
- Kitchen scales
- A ball pump

Take your basketball and, on the opposite side to the valve, cut a curved, hand-sized slit in it that resembles a smiling mouth. Pull the slit open and pour the sand or gravel in. A light- to moderate-weight medicine ball is 5 kg; a more serious weight is 10 kg. Use the rubber cement to glue the slot closed. Spread a layer of glue over the outside of the slit for reinforcement. Once the glue has hardened, stick a layer of duct tape over the slit and then pump the ball up. Don't pressurize the ball too much. Firstly, you may cause your repair to blow out and, secondly, a very hard medicine ball is no fun to use.

Your homemade medicine ball is suitable for lifting, throwing and catching exercises, but will not stand up to the rigours of full-blooded slams.

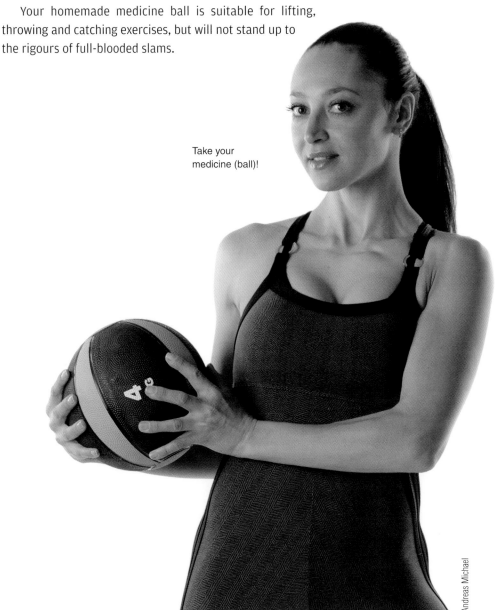

Take your
medicine (ball)!

Andreas Michael

CHAPTER FOUR

Cardio – getting to the heart (and lungs) of the matter

J ust about everyone knows that aerobic exercise is good for your heart and lungs (collectively called your cardiovascular system). As a general rule, the better conditioned your heart and lungs, the healthier these organs should be. The American College of Sports Medicine and other medical institutions all link cardio-vascular fitness to a reduced incidence of high blood pressure, coronary heart disease, heart attack and stroke. Cardiovascular exercise is also important for weight control and improving sports performance.

In an effort to further emphasize the importance of cardiovascular fitness, let's take a look at your innards and learn a little more about what is going on inside your chest cavity right now...

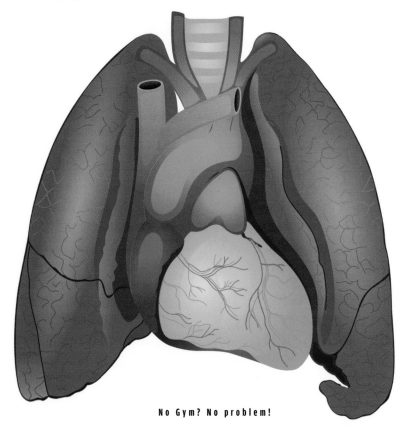

Heart and lungs – out of sight but never out of mind

Dreamstime.com

Every breath you take…

It's likely that the only time you think about breathing is when you can't (!), e.g. after a hard interval training session or when forgetting to breathe during a set of press-ups. Breathing is a purely involuntary process that, at rest, happens an average of twelve times per minute and is controlled by the autonomic nervous system, which ensures our bodies get a steady supply of oxygen 24/7.

Chemoreceptors (chemical sensing organs) detect levels of carbon dioxide in the blood and concentrations reach a critical level as you breathe. Inhalation (breathing in) occurs when the diaphragm and muscles in between the ribs (called the inter-costals) contract to expand the ribcage, which results in air being drawn into your lungs – just like a set of bellows. Air passes down the pharynx, larynx, trachea, bronchus, bronchi and bronchioles before reaching the alveoli, where the oxygen diffuses into the blood via microscopic blood vessels called capillaries, to then be circulated around your body. Exhalation (breathing out) is the action of the diaphragm and intercostals relaxing back into their original resting position, which drives air out of the lungs. We can also use the muscles of the abdomen to 'squeeze' air out when we need to breathe out more forcefully than usual.

As you exercise, your need for oxygen naturally increases and subsequently your breathing rate increases. During very intense exercise your breathing rate can rise to as many as forty-five breaths per minute in healthy, fit individuals.

And the beat goes on…

Just like your car has a fuel pump, we have a blood pump called the myocardium or heart in plain English! The heart is a four-chambered muscle that can be divided into two halves - the left side and the right side. The left side of the heart is respon-sible for the pumping of oxygenated blood around the body and the right side pumps deoxygenated blood back into the lungs. When describing the heart, left and right are reversed, as if you were describing the heart of someone facing you. The upper chambers of the heart are the receiving chambers and are called the atria (atrium = singular) and the lower chambers of the heart are the ejecting cham-bers and are called ventricles.

Blood vessels called veins take blood towards the heart whilst arteries take blood away. Blood flows from atrium to ventricle and blood is prevented from flowing back-wards by one-way valves called atrioventricular valves (AV valves for short).

The average resting heart rate is seventy-two beats per minute although this can be lowered significantly in very fit people. It is not uncommon for well-condi-tioned endurance athletes to have resting heart rates of forty beats per minute or less. Your heart rhythm is controlled by a biological pacemaker - a bundle of nerves called the sinoatrial node or SAN. The heart, like the lungs, is an involuntary organ under the control of the autonomic nervous system, which responds to the demands of the body. If more oxygen is required, greater energy expenditure is necessary, or if you are feeling stressed or scared, the heart will speed up to match your body's demands.

Blood pressure

Blood pressure describes the force that the blood exerts against the artery walls and is a major indicator of health. The harder your heart beats, the higher the blood volume there is or the greater the resistance to blood flow there is, the higher the blood pressure will be. Your blood pressure is measured in millimetres of mercury (mmHg) and is divided into two readings – an upper figure called systolic blood pressure and a lower figure called diastolic blood pressure. Systolic blood pressure describes blood pressure as the heart is contracting (beating) whilst diastolic blood pressure describes blood pressure when the heart is relaxed.

Blood pressure is measured using a sphygmomanometer or blood-pressure cuff and the accepted norm is 140/80 mmHg. Readings below this are referred to as hypotension and anything above as hypertension (this may need medical attention). Hypertension puts significant stress on organs such as the kidneys and the heart and has numerous causes; stress, excess dietary salt, a sedentary lifestyle, smoking, obesity, blocked arteries and excess fluid retention can all contribute to elevated blood pressure. The good news is that exercise and a healthy diet can go a long way to keeping blood pressure levels normal. Because hypertension has no external symptoms, it's very important to check your blood pressure regularly to avoid any unseen problems developing.

Gauging intensity

So now you know a little about how your heart and lungs work, we need to discuss how to get them as fit, well-conditioned and healthy as possible without the use of lots of fancy, expensive exercise equipment.

As I have said before, improvements in fitness are positive adaptations to stress. This means that you have to overload the systems of your body if you want to get fitter. If there is too little or too much stress your body will not adapt, so it's important to gauge the intensity of your workouts for maximum results. After all, if you go to all the bother of getting up early to exercise you want the best fitness return for your time and effort investment, don't you?!

Use these handy tools to monitor your exercise intensity and make sure your workouts hit the 'sweet spot' of being as effective as possible:

Breathing pattern
When you perform aerobic exercise such as jogging or rowing, your muscles use

more oxygen and produce carbon dioxide. Carbon-dioxide levels are monitored by chemoreceptors in your blood vessels, which send messages to your lungs via your brain to increase the speed and depth of your breathing. As you increase the intensity of your workout, you switch from nose breathing to mouth breathing. This is (or was, because now you'll be looking for it!) an automatic response to the increased demand for oxygen and occurs at around sixty per cent of your maximum heart rate. The bottom line is that, if you are breathing through your nose when doing your cardio, you're probably not working hard enough.

Appearance

Like a bad gambler, you have an exercise 'tell'. You may go red, sweat at a certain exercise intensity, develop an intense 'thousand-yard stare', clench your fists or exhibit a host of other signs when you hit your training sweet spot. Once you know what your tells are, you can use them to monitor the intensity of your workout. These tells, like the breathing mentioned earlier, are a subconscious indicator of how you are feeling but, now, because you are aware of them, you need to relax and just let them happen.

Talk test

Talking is reliant on your ability to breathe, specifically to exhale. As you already know, when you exercise your breathing rate increases as your need for oxygen increases. The faster your breathing rate, the harder it is to talk. The next time you are working out, try chatting to a friend and monitor your speech patterns. If you can tell them where you are going for your holiday, what you are going to pack, the time of your flight and the colour of your swimsuit without pausing for breath you probably aren't working hard enough! If, however, you are reduced to monosyllabic words and grunts, you are probably working too hard ... certainly beyond your anaerobic threshold. One or two breaths per sentence would suggest that you are working aerobically and will get plenty of benefit from your workout.

Rating of perceived exertion

Attributed to Swede Gunner Borg, the Rating of Perceived Exertion scale, or RPE for short, is a method of monitoring intensity based on how you feel while exercising. Borg's original scale runs from six to twenty, which may seem a little odd, but Borg was working with very fit athletes who, on average, had a resting heart rate of around 60 bpm and a maximum heart rate of 200 bpm. By knocking off a zero, he devised a scale that was linked to heart rate but didn't actually require his athletes to monitor their pulses. Instead of working at, for example, 140 bpm, Borg would have his athletes exercise at level fourteen.

RPE level	How does it feel?
6	Rest
7	Very, very light
8	
9	Very light
10	
11	Fairly light
12	
13	Somewhat hard – steady pace
14	
15	Hard
16	
17	Very hard
18	
18	Very, very hard
20	Maximum effort

With practice, using Borg's scale can be very precise, but some users find the concept of a six to twenty scale offputting and, as a result, a modified version of Borg's scale emerged with numbers from one to ten. Many users find this modified scale far more logical and user-friendly. If you wish to correlate heart rate with this modified scale, you can make the assumption that level six is equal to around sixty of your maximum heart rate.

RPE level	How does it feel?	% of MHR
1	At rest	10
2	Very easy	20
3	Moderate – can talk easily	30
4	More purposeful – breathing is faster	40
5	Starting to become warm – sporadic conversation	50
6	Challenging but sustainable for 20 minutes or more	60
7	Very challenging – short sentences only	70
8	Very tough – one word answers only	80
9	Almost flat out	90
10	Absolute limit – maximum heart rate, only sustainable for a few seconds	100

When I explain this scale to my clients, I tell them that 'level one is equal to being sat at home, feet up, watching TV, whilst level ten is sprinting after a bus that just won't stop' and I encourage them to find level five or six. By combining the talk test, observing breathing patterns and using RPE, I can get my clients to sixty per cent of their heart-rate training zone (the range in which your heart rate should remain while exercising) without having to use a heart-rate monitor.

The main disadvantage with both scales of perceived exertion is that they do not take into account exercise discomfort tolerance. If you find a particular activity uncomfortable, you will probably perceive that you are working harder than you actually are.

Heart rate

Your heart drives blood around your body. The harder you exercise, the greater the demand for oxygenated blood, and therefore the higher your heart rate will be. Because your heart responds to exercise in a very predictable way, you can use your heart rate to monitor exercise intensity. You can measure your heart rate by using a heart-rate monitor, taking your pulse at your wrist or neck or using the sensors built into cardio exercise equipment.

To get the most from your aerobic exercise, you should stay between sixty to ninety per cent of your maximum heart rate. Exercising below sixty per cent means that the stress placed on your body will likely be insufficient to trigger much in the way of fitness improvements whereas working above ninety per cent takes your exercise intensity towards the point where your body switches from aerobic energy

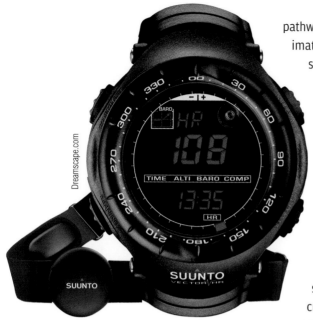

Dreamscape.com

Heart-rate monitors can be a useful way to monitor your workout intensity

pathways to anaerobic. While anaerobic exercise is a legitimate form of training, for most people it's unnecessarily demanding and, to be honest, you don't need to know your heart rate to know you are working above your anaerobic threshold; your burning muscles, heaving chest and desire to stop will let you know in no uncertain terms!

There are a number of ways you can calculate your heart-rate training zone...

Karvonan method

The most common method for calculating heart-rate training zone is called the Karvonan method. The Karvonan method is very simple and this simplicity is one of the reasons this method has its critics. To calculate your heart-rate training zone, perform the following calculation:

- 220 – your age in years = maximum heart rate
- 60% of maximum heart rate = lower end of your training zone
- 90% of maximum heart rate = upper end of your training zone

Example for a 35-year-old:
- 220 - 35 = 185 MHR
- 60% of 185 = 111 bpm
- 90% of 185 = 166.5 bpm

Critics of the Karvonan method believe that this formula does not reflect the needs of individual exercisers or take into account current fitness levels. I had a client whose ninety per cent figure was 165 bpm but was comfortable exercising at 200 bpm and had an actual maximum heart rate of 215 bpm. However, for some people, including me, the Karvonan method provides an appropriate training zone for aerobic exercise.

Heart Rate Reserve

A second, more personalized method for calculating your heart-rate training zone is called Heart Rate Reserve or HRR. Heart Rate Reserve tends to result in a higher heart-rate training zone when compared with the Karvonan method and is popular with endurance athletes. To use this calculation, you need to know your resting heart rate. Obtain this figure by taking your heart rate when you are relaxed, well rested and caffeine free.

Example for a 35-year-old with a resting heart rate of 60 bpm:

- 220 - 60 - 35 = 125
- 60% of 125 + 60 = 135 bpm
- 90% of 125 + 60 = 172.5 bpm

As you can see, HRR results in a higher training zone than the basic Karvonan method calculation for the same exerciser.

Maximum heart-rate tests

Maximal heart-rate tests are stressful but, providing you have the drive to push yourself as hard as possible, they will provide an accurate figure with which you can calculate your personalized heart-rate training zone. It goes without saying that you should only perform a maximal heart-rate test if you are fit, healthy, experienced and injury-free and then only after a thorough warm-up.

There are a number of ways you can achieve a maximum heart rate, including the following workouts and tests...

- Four-minute maximum effort run/row
- Two to three 400 m intervals with thirty to sixty seconds of recovery
- Multi-stage fitness test (a.k.a. the bleep test)
- Incremental treadmill test (increase incline and/or speed every minute until you have to stop)

Each test should end with you feeling that you couldn't have run any faster or further and that you just HAD to stop. Anything less than a maximal effort will fail to produce a maximum heart rate. Because you will be exhausted at the end of the test and your heart rate will drop quickly on completion, you should wear a heart-rate monitor to ensure you get an accurate reading – you won't want to have to repeat the test any time soon! Once you have your maximum heart rate, calculate sixty and ninety per cent to determine your personalized heart-rate training zone.

Cardiovascular training modalities for the home exerciser

Running

Of all the ways you can exercise your heart and lungs, running is probably the most easily accessible. To experience the benefits of running all you really need are some suitable shoes and access to the great outdoors. Whether you choose to pound the pavements or get out into the countryside, there is no denying that running is an effective way to get in great shape.

So, does this mean that everyone should run? Absolutely not. I have a long and

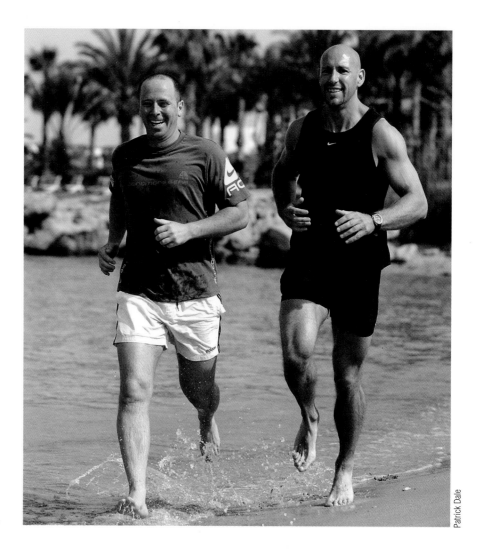

Running – effective
but not for everyone

Patrick Dale

varied history of running. I have competed at a high level in everything from 5 km to half-marathon distance, was a successful triathlete, ran a great deal in my career as a Marine and now, despite those thirty or so years of running, seldom run and never for more than a few 400 m intervals. Why? Well, after years of hard training I have arthritic knees that really don't respond well to the repeated impact of long-distance running. I tried a 'comeback' twelve months ago, but within a few short weeks of light training I was reduced to walking with a limp. My distance running days are over except for the occasional jog on the beach where the sand helps to absorb much of the injurious impact.

Lots of people have long and enjoyable running careers but this doesn't mean that everyone should try and emulate them. If you are a bit on the heavy side (muscle or fat weight), have a history of lower limb or back pain, are a female with an above-average width pelvis or simply don't enjoy running, don't worry; running

No Gym? No problem!

is not compulsory for fitness. Cardio is all but essential but if running doesn't suit you (or you don't suit running) then there are plenty of alternative and equally effective cardiovascular training methods for you to try.

Although running appears to be a simple undertaking, if you choose to make it part of your workouts you should endeavour to make it as enjoyable, safe and beneficial as possible by following these simple tips:

Wear the right shoes – the way you run, commonly referred to as your gait, can have a huge impact on your running performance and the likelihood of suffering long-term injuries. Your gait is likely to fall into one of five main categories:

- **Pronated** – meaning your feet roll inwards towards your big toe
- **Supinated** – known as under-pronation and meaning your feet roll outwards towards your little toe
- **Neutral** – meaning your feet roll normally you
- **Heel striking** – meaning you tend to land heavily on your heels
- **Forefoot striking** – meaning you tend to land more on the balls of your feet

A specialist running-shoe fitter should be able to identify your running gait, which often differs from your walking gait, and recommend shoes that will offer the cushioning and support appropriate to your needs. The right shoes can make all the difference and significantly reduce your chances of suffering chronic running-related injuries such as ankle, knee and hip problems. While you don't need to spend a fortune on running shoes, spend enough to ensure you have a shoe that matches your running gait.

You can assess your own gait simply by looking at your current running shoes. Notable wear on the outside of your shoe suggests you are a supinator whereas wear on the inside of your shoe suggests you are a pronator.

You may have noticed a trend towards so-called minimalist running shoes that provide zero cushioning or support in an effort to make you run as though you were barefoot. While it may be true that running barefoot means the muscles of your feet and calves will have to work harder and behave in a more natural fashion compared with their behaviour in a more engineered shoe, the fact of the matter is that years and years of wearing shoes has left us very reliant on cushioned and supportive footwear.

Hopping onto the barefoot bandwagon (pun intended!) and doing too much too soon is likely to cause as many problems as these shoes are supposed to cure, so if you do decide to try the *au naturel* approach to running, start slowly and build up very gradually. I suggest running for no more than five minutes every other day and applying the ten per cent rule to subsequent increases in mileage - see page 64.

Running barefoot promotes a mid- to forefoot strike, compared to the heel strike promoted by regular running shoes. While this does make more use of the natural shock-absorbing mechanisms in your foot, it is also a very unusual movement for most of us. Jumping from heel striking to forefoot/toe striking is likely to result in very sore arches and calves and a severe case of Achilles tendonitis.

Our barefoot-running ancestors, the inspiration for minimalist shoes, always had strong feet and ankles, so they never had to worry about making the transition from wearing shoes to running shoeless. Our soft and pandered feet, however, have been coddled since birth so it'll take some time for them to become accustomed to running in the nude, so to speak!

Don't run in 'dead' shoes – even the best running shoe is only good for around 500 mi before the support and cushioning, so important for keeping you free of injuries and running comfortably, starts to break down. A low mileage or occasional runner could get almost a year out of a pair of shoes but a marathon runner in heavy training may need to replace their shoes every two months.

Also, remember that, by and large, runners are slender folk who carry little in the way of excess bodyweight. And that's who many top-range running shoes are designed for. If, in reality, you are a bit on the beefy side then it's important to realize that your running shoes are going to suffer more punishment and should be replaced more often as a result.

It's all too easy to become emotionally attached to your current running shoes but once they begin to break down, your best friend can become your worst enemy. If you find a make and model of shoe you really *really* like, consider buying multiple pairs and wearing them in rotation. As one pair 'dies' you can replace them, safe in the knowledge that you don't have to swap brands. For many years I only ever wore one make and model of shoe and always bought multiple pairs. What seems like an extravagance can actually save you a lot of money in physiotherapy bills.

Follow the ten per cent rule – imagine you are running three times a week and each run covers 3 mi. Your weekly mileage works out at 9 mi. After a few weeks, and adhering quite rightly to the rule of overload discussed back in Chapter 2 (see pages 16-17), you decide to up your mileage to 4 mi per run. That single extra mile per run bumps your weekly training mileage by twenty-five per cent. That's a sizable increase.

Most running experts agree that such large jumps in training mileage or running frequency tend to lead to an increased occurrence of running-related injuries. Remember, running is exercise and exercise is a form of stress. A little stress is good – actually, essential – however, too much too soon can be detrimental to your long-term health. Most running injuries: shin splints, runner's knee, Achilles tendonitis to name but three, are normally insidious and are linked to asking too much from your body too soon.

In most cases, the only remedy to these types of injury is a break from all running and then, after possibly months of rest, a very gradual and tentative return. Avoid these chronic injuries by only increasing your weekly running mileage by ten per cent per week. This is slow progress but will add up to big improvements over the coming months.

Look after your feet – unsurprisingly, running is hard on your feet. Corns, hard skin, ingrown toenails and athlete's foot can all make what should be an enjoyable experience much less so. Make sure you keep your feet in good working order by wearing the right shoes (but then you know that already), wearing good quality running socks, keeping your nails trimmed short but not brutally so, drying properly between your toes, using surgical tape on known 'hot spots' if you are prone to blisters and even consider a monthly pedicure to give your feet a well-deserved MOT. A minor foot complaint, such as a blister, can alter the way you run, which can throw stress onto an unaccustomed joint or muscle and result in an injury. Be nice to your feet and they'll be nice to you – a lesson I learnt the hard way in the Marines!

Be seen – motorists tend to be a bit blind to runners, especially as runners can and often do dodge in and out of traffic in an effort to beat their best training times. Don't become one of the growing numbers of runner/car collision statistics. Take care around traffic, make sure you wear bright and/or reflective clothing for maximum visibility and remember to run defensively. Always assume the driver hasn't seen you and act accordingly. You might well be in the right in an altercation with a car but, right or not, it will be you who comes off the worst.

Also if, like me, you like to exercise while using an MP3 player, take extra care when running in the streets. Your hearing can provide an early warning of approaching automotive danger and blocking that sense with music means you are more at risk of suffering an accident. If you do use an MP3 or similar music player while out running, keep the volume low enough to hear approaching traffic.

Learn how to run – I'm sure you think you know how to run but do you really run in the most effective and efficient way? Do you float across the ground hardly leaving any footprints or do you stomp it to a powder? Are your footfalls light and all but silent or do herds of elephants cover their ears when you run past!? Is your upper body relaxed and do you flow from one step to the next like water over a waterfall or do you look like a heavyweight wrestler running full speed through knee-deep molasses even though you are just warming up? You get the idea...

Running coaching can help cure these and many other running-related maladies. Good running technique is energy efficient so you'll go further and faster for the same energy output, and it is also less stressful so you should suffer fewer running-related injuries. An effective running technique converts more of your energy into forward momentum and helps take the brakes off. Getting fitter is only part of the running faster equation.

Swimming

I was unsure whether to include swimming in this book as, unless you are fortunate enough to have a swimming pool in your garden, it doesn't really fit with the home-training ethos. On reflection though, its inclusion is warranted because swimming, it could be argued, is actually more no-frills then running.

Unless you are an exhibitionist skinny-dipper, all you need for swimming is a pair of goggles and a swimming costume. As most towns have at least one swimming pool you should have no problem finding a suitable venue.

So what is suitable? In my early triathlon days, I trained in a 17-m long pool, which was far from ideal, but that was what I had access to. Swimming just less than one hundred lengths to a mile can really make you good at turns (and counting!) but a 20-m or longer pool is really a much better choice.

Swimming is not just low-impact, it is no-impact. This makes it ideal if you are overweight, suffer from lower limb or back pain or just want a joint-friendly workout. The water supports your bodyweight so, while swimming can deliver an effective workout, it does so without placing an inordinate amount of stress on your body.

Swimming – an essential life skill and a great form of exercise

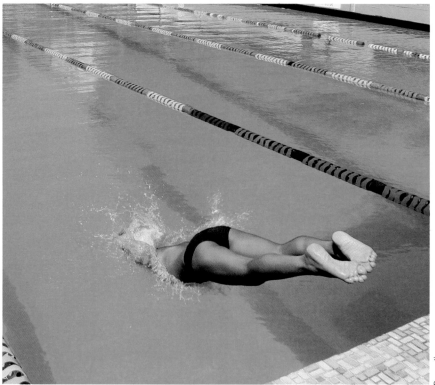

Dreamstime.com

On the downside, to get a good workout from swimming you need to be able to swim! If one width of the pool is all you can manage, swimming is not going to elevate your heart rate for long enough for you to experience much in the way of cardiovascular benefit. Ideally you need to be able to swim for twenty minutes at a time at a reasonably steady pace to experience much in the way of improved fitness. Learning to swim this far can take time but with perseverance and possibly some coaching most people can become competent enough to be able to swim for exercise.

The key to swimming is technique. Water is much denser than air so you need to try and carve through it like a hot knife through butter. Poor aqua-dynamics means that each metre you swim will take more effort because of increased water resistance. The more resistance there is the more energy you'll expend, the slower you will travel and, most likely, the sooner you will need to stop.

Learning to swim smoothly and economically means your energy will be used predominately to drive you forwards through the water rather than merely thrashing the water to foam.

In terms of stroke, in theory any stroke will do but having swum a lot as a triathlete, front crawl, which is also known as freestyle, is probably your best choice. The elongated body position and low profile in the water means that front crawl allows you to travel further, faster and for less effort. Learning to breathe is probably the hardest part of freestyle swimming but, once mastered, will mean that you should be able to swim rings around even a decent breaststroke swimmer. The appeal of breaststroke is that you can perform it with your head out of the water. This may be attractive if you are nervous about putting your face in the water but the high chest/low legs position common in breaststroke means that there is a lot of drag to overcome and that means that breaststroke is not really suitable for serious fitness swimming.

Equipment-wise, and in addition to your swimming costume and goggles, there are a few simple tools that can help you hone your swimming technique and also provide some workout variety...

- **Pull buoys** – looking like a three-dimensional figure of eight, a pull buoy is designed to be held between your legs to provide lower-body buoyancy and allow you to focus on your arm action.
- **Kick boards** – the traditional swimmer's float, the kick board is held in your hands so you can only use your legs to produce thrust. A few lengths of legs-only swimming will soon show you whether you have a kick like a motorboat outboard engine or are merely dragging them behind you like so much useless dead weight.
- **Fins** – training fins are smaller than snorkelling/diving fins and are designed to increase the surface area of your feet. This makes kicking harder and

subsequently increases your kicking power. Swimming legs-only while wearing fins is the swimming equivalent of hill repeats when running or cycling, especially when combined with using a kick board.

- **Aqua gloves** – these webbed gloves allow you to 'grab' more water and increase the amount of power you can generate with your arms. This increases the overload on your upper-body muscles. Aqua gloves are an effective training aid that can really help you develop a better feel for the water.
- **Buoyancy aids** – not for life preservation, these foam belts will help keep you afloat and, more importantly, vertical in deep water. This allows you to 'run' through the water, which is why these devices are also known as aqua jogging belts. The action of running in deep water can help maintain running fitness when injury prevents you from pounding the pavement. Deep water running is also a great way to get some water-based exercise even if you are not an especially strong swimmer.
- **Drag suits** – not as kinky as they sound, drag suits are like regular swimming costumes but have specially made pockets attached to the outside that act like mini parachutes and increase your drag through the water. This is a great way to overload your swimming muscles and cardiovascular system and can help 'level the playing field' if you swim with someone less capable than yourself.

Here are some tips to help you get the most out of your swimming workouts...

- Public pools can be very crowded and nothing will ruin your flow more than having to dodge people swimming widths while you are swimming lengths. Try to swim when the pool is divided into lanes so you can focus on ploughing up and down in a straight line rather than zig-zagging.
- Join a swimming club. Swimming clubs offer structured workouts and coaching and also the potential for a competitive outlet for your fitness. Beginners are always welcome and many clubs offer masters' (older) swimming sessions as well as beginners' and improvers' lessons
- Don't just swim; train. Swimming is great exercise but only if you go into the water with a plan and swim with determination and effort. Floating aimlessly about for thirty minutes or so won't do much for your fitness! Instead, break your workout down into a warm-up, technique drills using kick boards, pull buoys etc., a main session consisting of intervals or any of the other training systems described elsewhere in this book and, finally, a cool-down.
- Learn a variety of strokes and use them to break up your workout. Different strokes use different muscle groups and while front crawl/freestyle should be your 'go to' stroke, breaststroke, backstroke and even butterfly all have their place. Use these strokes in your warm-up and cool-down as well as your active rests between harder bouts of swimming freestyle.

- Don't neglect hydration. Although you probably don't realize it, you lose water when you are swimming. Exhaled air contains a lot of water (in the form of vapour), and you'll also sweat, although it is washed away instantly. Take a plastic or otherwise unbreakable bottle with you and drink as you would during any land-based workout.

Even if you choose not to swim for exercise, swimming is an all but essential skill that could one day help save your life or the life of another. If you can't swim, consider joining one of the many adult 'learn to swim' classes that are part of most local authorities' swimming pool schedules.

Cycling

Cycling is great exercise, not least because, as a low-impact activity, it is suitable for heavier exercisers and those with other impact-related lower limb injuries. On the downside, you obviously need a bike to enjoy the cardiovascular benefits offered by cycling.

You can cycle for fitness on just about any kind of bike; mountain, road or hybrid. Each has advantages and disadvantages so it's really a case of either making do with what you've got or selecting a bike based on the type of cycling you are going to do most...

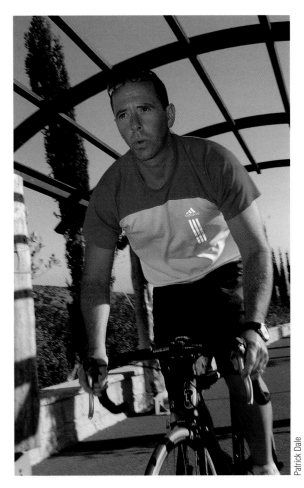

Patrick Dale

Cycling is a great way to maintain or increase cardiovascular fitness

Mountain bikes

With the exception of top-price models, mountain bikes tend to be heavier than road bikes. This is because they are made to be tough and durable so they can survive the rigours of riding off-road. Most mountain bikes offer a large number of gears so you can conquer almost any incline and the upright riding position can make for a more comfortable ride, as well as making it easier to look ahead without getting neck-ache. However, this upright position is less aerodynamic so you'll have to work harder to reach high speeds than on a more low-profile road bike.

Suspension, a feature of many mountain bikes, is great if you are going to spend a lot of time off-road, but the flexibility of the frame and/or forks will also absorb a significant part of your pedalling energy and mean that you will lose some speed on the road.

If you intend to use your mountain bike on the road, it's worth considering fitting it with low-profile road tyres to minimize rolling resistance. Road tyres are much smoother than knobbly off-road tyres and will allow you to go further and faster for less effort. There are also tyres designed for mixed terrain – another good option.

Mountain bikes tend to feel very stable because of the riding position and smaller, wider wheels compared to a road bike and are a good choice for novice or occasional cyclists.

Road bikes

As the name suggests, road bikes are designed to be ridden on the road. They are characterized by their narrow tyres, 'drop' handlebars and bent-over riding position. The aerodynamic riding position, combined with a generally lighter machine, means that road bikes tend to be faster than mountain bikes although obviously this ultimately depends on the fitness of the rider. Some cyclists initially find riding in a tucked position uncomfortable. To limit this you should make sure your bike is set up properly and the handlebars are not too low. Also, make sure your frame is the right size for you and, if you are serious about cycling, consider getting a custom-frame made so the bike geometry is matched to your unique body shape.

Road bikes are normally fitted with very smooth tyres to maximize speed. The narrow wheels reduce road contact and therefore friction. While narrow wheels and smooth tyres can enhance speed, they also mean that a road bike is out of its element on anything other than smooth roads in good condition. Hitting a pothole at 20 mph is very likely to destroy a road bike wheel whereas a mountain bike will probably just bounce over it.

If covering long distances at speed is your aim, a road bike is probably your best choice, but if you ride on rough roads or are considering riding off-road, a mountain bike is a better option.

Hybrid bikes

Sometimes called commuter bikes, hybrids are the successful marriage of road bikes and mountain bikes. Basically a mountain-bike frame with larger, low-profile wheels, hybrids are popular with courier riders as they are fast, agile, comfortable and tough; not as tough as a fully-fledged mountain bike but certainly up to the challenge of even the most poorly maintained roads.

A hybrid bike is ideal if you want an upright riding position but don't want to completely lose on-road performance. While definitely faster than a typical mountain bike (again, depending on the fitness of the rider) the comfortable upright riding position will increase your aerodynamic drag so bear this in mind if speed is one of your cycling requirements.

Added extras and precautions

In addition to a bike, there are a few items and precautions that can help make your cycling as enjoyable, safe and productive as possible...

- **Buy and learn to use clipless pedals/shoes** – regular exercise shoes are fine for a spin down to the shops but all that spongy shock absorbency will soak up some of your pedalling effort and waste valuable energy. Also, cycling quickly and efficiently is more than just stamping downwards on your pedals; you should also be pushing forwards, pulling back and pulling up. This means you need to be attached to your pedals. Being fixed to your bike takes some getting used to so don't venture out into traffic until you are completely comfortable with your shoe and pedal connection. The last thing you want to do is pull up at a set of traffic lights and then find you can't disengage your foot from the pedal. Falling down in the street is seldom cool.

- **Dress to impress** – I don't mean impress in terms of fashion, more in terms of comfort and visibility. If you spend long enough on a bike, you'll soon understand why cycling shorts are made with reinforced seats that are generally padded. In the old days, which I sadly remember, the pads in cycling shorts were made of chamois leather, which meant you couldn't wash your shorts and had to wax the leather pad to keep it supple. Thankfully, short pads are now made from synthetic and washing machine-friendly materials so you don't have to worry about smelling like something has died in your underpants. Cycling shorts don't have to mean figure-hugging Lycra; you can also get cargo/skateboard-style cycling shorts that wouldn't look out of place on the beach. As for the rest of your cycling wardrobe, just dress for the elements as you would with any outdoor workout, but remember that wind chill plays a role when pedalling along at a decent pace and, while your legs may stay warm, your feet, hands and head/face can get painfully cold very quickly. Overshoes, gloves and a hat are all but essential clothing items for cold weather cycling.

- **Wear a helmet** – bones mend, brains don't, or so the saying goes. Sadly, in almost every case, it's the cyclist who will end up injured in a collision with another vehicle – even if they are 'in the right'. It's all too easy to fall off if you hit wet leaves or an oily patch on the road. Protect your most vital organ by always wearing a helmet designed specifically for cycling. Modern helmets are light, well ventilated and very effective at directing impact forces away from your fragile skull and brain. Do not skimp on this vital piece of equipment!

- **Carry a repair kit** – punctures and mechanical problems can be a pain. I remember triumphantly overtaking a slow-moving lorry, complete with a contemptuous look back over my shoulder, only to get a puncture 200 m down the road and then have to a) see the lorry pass me again and b) push my crippled bike home as I had no puncture repair kit on me. Learn from my mistakes by not gloating when you overtake slow-moving traffic and always carrying a rudimentary repair kit with you so you can fix a puncture, adjust your gears or carry out any other emergency repairs that will allow you to make your way home.

- **Be traffic aware** – courier riders are notoriously foolhardy and weave in and out of traffic with what seems like complete disregard for their safety. More often than not they leave a trail of angry motorists in their wake, but it's okay – they are professional riders just doing their job. Actually, it's not okay but, just because many bike messengers seem to have delusions of immortality, it doesn't mean you need to ride like they do. Even with your compulsory helmet firmly in place, you are literally putting your life on the line if you fail to observe the rules of the road. So, and at the risk of sounding like an overly strict parent, please do not jump traffic lights, ride on the pavement, ride without lights at night, forget your high-visibility jacket, wear a MP3 player or any other device that will stop you hearing the approach of traffic, ride aggressively or provocatively. If I had to sum up how to cycle safely, I would use the phrase 'ride defensively'. Always be on your guard and assume motorists have not seen you approaching. Do that and you'll reduce your risk of suffering an accident.

I've ridden bikes my whole life and have owned some really top-quality machines – both road and mountain bikes. As a triathlete I frequently rode 150 mi a week come rain or shine and, while I never raced any of my mountain bikes, I covered a lot of miles on them, on- and off-road. I've also commuted on my bikes – 15 mi to Bath from Bristol every day, five days a week for two years, and more recently 5 mi each way into the centre of Paphos and back – downhill going and uphill coming back. I've had a long and rewarding love affair with cycling and bikes in general and I think that, if you have the time (bike rides tend to be longer than other comparable workouts – although they can be a useful way to turn your daily commute into a workout) and the inclination, cycling is a great way to develop your fitness.

Cardiovascular exercise machines

Just because you choose to train at home doesn't mean you can't have access to one or some of the cardiovascular machines so typical of modern gyms. There are lots of companies selling light-commercial or home-use equipment designed to do more or less the same job as the 'real' workout equipment for a considerably lower price. While there is an abundance of this type of equipment available to choose from, there is a downside: home-use equipment is, by and large, less robust than commercial gym equipment.

That being said, if you hunt around, are prepared to haggle hard and even walk away if the price isn't right, you should be able to find some good bargains should you want to acquire some home-use cardio equipment. Also, there is an abundance of second-hand training equipment available to buy on the internet and in newspapers and magazines. Lots of people buy this type of equipment with the best of intentions and then find they simply don't use it. (Don't be one of them!) A friend of mine recently picked up a commercial-quality rower, hardly used, for less than half price.

Exercise bikes

While cycling outdoors is great exercise, it's not without drawbacks. Bad weather, heavy traffic and not having a bike (!) can all put a cramp on your cycling ambitions. An indoor exercise bike may be the answer. There are numerous styles of exercise bikes. Some use a large electromagnet to provide pedalling resistance while others use a simple flywheel and belt system. Alternatively, you can buy rollers and a device called a 'turbo trainer' that will convert your regular bike into an exercise machine. I used a turbo trainer a lot in my triathlon training as it provided an excellent way to perform intervals in a safe and easily quantifiable environment. Park your bike in front of the TV and simply spin away. A major plus-side for exercise bikes is that they are very quiet to use, which makes them ideal if you have thin walls or neighbours with good hearing!

Cross-trainers

Using a cross-trainer involves performing a stepping/skiing leg action and, often, an alternating arm action as well. They provide an effective low impact workout and are also relatively quiet to use. Abiding by the rule of specificity, cross-trainers develop a very specific type of fitness; in other words, frequent use of a cross-trainer will make you good at using a cross-trainer! If you are looking for an activity to augment your running or cycling workouts then you need to look at exercise bikes and treadmills, but if you are more interested in improving your general conditioning, a cross-trainer is a good choice, especially one with an arm action.

Treadmills

As discussed earlier, running (and indeed walking) are probably the most natural ways to develop cardiovascular fitness. As running requires no equipment other than a decent pair of shoes and can be performed just about anywhere, it really is hard to find another activity that offers so many benefits in such a simple package. Some people, however, prefer to do their running on a treadmill rather than outside. A good commercial treadmill is a big machine with a powerful motor and large running deck. They are generally pleasant to use and provide a quality workout. Light-commercial and home-use treadmills tend to have much smaller motors, a smaller running deck and aren't usually as sturdy. This may make your workout less than enjoyable. Unless you are going to buy a reasonably high-quality machine with a decent top speed and variable incline, personally, I'd stick to running outdoors. If you do decide you want a treadmill, bear in mind they are generally quite noisy, are not usually portable and take up a lot of space.

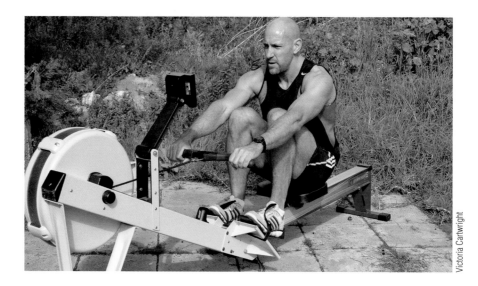

Victoria Cartwright

Rowing machines –
not cheap but more
portable than a
treadmill

Rowing machines

Rowing machines offer a total-body, low-impact workout but are also low impact,
which makes them ideal for heavier exercisers or those of us whose knees aren't up
to the repetitive impact of running. Like all of the aforementioned cardiovascular
equipment, there are good rowers and bad ones. The better ones use large fans
for resistance, while the not-so-good ones use hydraulic levers. I have a rowing
machine in my garage and it is my 'go to' cardio workout for home use. While it is
not especially quiet to use, the fact that it's a non-impact exercise means you won't
disturb your neighbours and, while it is quite long, many models can simply be
stood upright and tucked away in a corner. There is very little that can go wrong
with a rowing machine and they tend to be very hard-wearing. Mine is over five
years old, gets used outdoors a lot and has never broken down. On the downside,
if indeed there is one, rowing does require a modicum of skill and rowing with bad
technique is likely to result in a sore lower back. If you do decide that rowing is for
you, please make sure you learn to row properly to get the most from your rower
and avoid any unnecessary injuries.

Considerations

I provide you with plenty of equipment-free cardio options in this
chapter and elsewhere in this book, so please don't feel under pressure to spend your hard-earned money on something that you will
only use occasionally and that might even end up merely doubling as
an expensive clothes horse! However, if you feel you've got the space,
the spare cash and the inclination, one or two well-chosen pieces of

cardiovascular equipment can be a great addition to your home gym. If you do decide you would like to purchase cardio equipment for home use, consider these following points...

- **Location** – where are you going to use your machine? For example, putting a treadmill anywhere where people will be below you is a bad idea because of the repetitive pounding.
- **Space** – consider the dimensions of the equipment. Exercise bikes tend to have the smallest 'footprint' while treadmills and rowers are much bigger. Make sure your chosen equipment will fit comfortably into your intended training space.
- **Spares** – are spare parts readily available? That cheap piece of equipment might not seem such a bargain if it breaks down and you can't replace a broken part. Check that the manufacturer is still operating and they hold a good stock of consumables.
- **Ventilation** – you are going to sweat heavily on your home cardio training equipment. Can you control the temperature of your training environment? If you have set your equipment up indoors, you really don't want to leave puddles of sweat on your carpet, so you may need to purchase fans to keep you cool and place matting on the floor beneath your machine. Commercial gyms have big air-conditioning units to keep exercisers cool; you probably do not.
- **Entertainment** – doing cardio at a gym means you have plenty to keep yourself amused while you work out: TV, piped music, chatting with friends or simply watching the comings and goings of your fellow gym users. Training at home can mean it's just you. If you get bored easily consider what you can do to keep yourself entertained while you work out. A well-placed TV, for example, can make an hour's workout fly by (and unlike at the gym you can choose the channel!). If nothing else, an MP3 player loaded with your favourite training music can make all the difference.
- **Quality** – remember, you get what you pay for and while there are bargains to be had if you look around, sometimes 'too good to be true' is exactly that! If your bargain exercise equipment is anything other than a joy to use, once the novelty factor wears off, you'll be left with something that merely gets in your way or is relegated to the back of your garage, never to be used again. If you can't afford to get something that will give you the workout you really want, save your money and buy a pair of decent running shoes and a skipping rope instead!

Circuit training

After running, cycling and swimming, you might be wondering what circuit training – usually thought of as a muscular endurance activity – is doing in my list of cardio-vascular training methods. Let me assure you, it didn't make it onto this list by mistake but because it is a very effective cardiovascular training method.

Circuit training involves performing a series of predetermined exercises back to back. The type and number of exercises are two of the many variables that can be manipulated to alter the intensity of the workout, but bodyweight exercises are a great choice and most circuits contain between four and twelve exercises.

Circuits can be repetition- or time-controlled. That is to say, you can perform a set number of repetitions per exercise, e.g. twenty, or perform each exercise for a set time, e.g. thirty seconds. Exercises are normally sequenced so that different muscle groups are worked from one exercise to the next. This means you can keep the workout intensity high while spreading the exercise stress around your body.

Here is a very simple circuit using bodyweight-only exercises. Notice how the exercises (all of which are detailed in the exercise library in Chapter 5) are sequenced to avoid overloading any one muscle group. Perform each exercise for thirty to sixty seconds, according to your fitness level, and rest for one to two minutes after completing the twelfth exercise. Repeat the entire sequence two or three more times.

1. Lunges
2. Press-ups
3. Crunches
4. Step-ups
5. Dips
6. Planks
7. Squats
8. 1½ side lateral raises
9. Seated Russian twist
10. Wrestler squats
11. Towel pull-downs
12. Sky divers

Circuit training provides a real double-whammy workout; you exercise every major muscle in your body (if you have designed a well-balanced circuit, that is!) and increase your cardiovascular fitness at the same time. Talk about workout efficiency! The effectiveness of circuit training is the reason many of the workouts in Chapter 8 are variations of circuit training. When it comes to getting a whole lot of exercise done in a relatively short time, circuit training is very hard to beat.

In addition to designing your own circuits and following the ones in this book, there are also lots of 'pay as you go' circuit-training classes around. Church halls, community centres, sports and recreation centres, parks and even beaches are all viable circuit-training venues.

When designing a circuit, you are only really limited by two things: the equipment you have available and your imagination. Space isn't an issue as you can literally train on the spot. No space to do shuttle runs? Sprint on the spot. No weights? Remember, your body is your gym. No timer? Count reps instead. Give me a 2 x 2 m space and I absolutely guarantee I can push you as hard as you have ever been pushed before without using any gym equipment. It won't be pretty, it won't be 'scientific', but I promise you will work hard despite being in what amounts to a prison cell. Try some of the workouts I've provided in Chapter 8 and then tell me it isn't so!

If you are short of time and want a 'does it all' workout, make circuit training part of your exercise regime.

Cardiovascular training methods

For many people, cardio is something they just 'turn up and do' with little in the way of planning. It's no wonder then that these same people fail to see much meaningful benefit from this type of exercise.

It's true that some of the benefit from cardio comes simply from being more active, but if you want to improve your cardiovascular fitness and performance you need to push the exercise envelope, move out of your comfort zone and train with purpose rather than simply rocking up, plugging in and switching off!

You can see 'no brainer' cardio training in action in gyms all around the country. Look for people who are happily plodding along at a sedate pace while reading a book or newspaper or busily updating their social-network status. While such a low level of intensity makes this kind of cardio enjoyable and accessible, it really won't do much for your fitness levels.

To get the most from your cardio training, both in terms of developing fitness and burning calories, it's vital that you consider the exercise law of overload. No overload equals no stimulus for adaptation; no adaptation equals a fitness plateau. Rather than doing the same old workouts week after week, month after month, make sure you look for ways to make your workouts progressively more challenging by manipulating the training variables detailed back in Chapter 2 (see pages 18–20). Also, periodically rotate your training methods to avoid a) boredom and b) fitness level stagnation.

Note – many of these training methods hail from running and so the associated terminology is often running-based. Don't let that put you off any of the methods. Each of the training techniques outlined below can be applied to pretty much any cardiovascular training modality. If a training method uses the term 'running', it's merely for illustrative purposes and you can just as easily cycle, swim, row or even skip. So long as you adhere to the principles of each method, you will get the results that each method is designed to deliver.

Long Slow Distance training

Called LSD for short, this type of training is what most people consider cardio to be. As the name suggests, LSD involves covering a relatively long distance at a slow and comfortable pace. Typically, an LSD workout is conducted at around sixty per cent of your age-adjusted maximum heart rate and at a pace where conversation is possible, your breathing rate is steady and you feel fairly comfortable.

LSD training, as the law of specificity suggests, increases your ability to run, cycle, swim or row a long way slowly. It improves your ability to work aerobically and develops basic aerobic fitness and muscular endurance. However, if you want to develop the ability to run faster and not just longer, you'll need to do more than simply plod mile after mile at a slow and steady speed. This type of workout is the cornerstone of many distance runner's training and rightly so. But, if you want to get more bang for your cardio buck, LSD should make up only a relatively small amount of your total weekly training volume.

In LSD training, your main exercise variable is duration. In other words, as the weeks go by, you should endeavour to increase the distance you travel or the duration of your workout. This is okay up to a point but what if, after months or even years of diligently increasing the length of your workouts, you find you can continue exercising for hours at a time? This is the main drawback with LSD training; at some point you will reach the point of diminishing returns and rather than see a marked improvement in your fitness, you'll hit a plateau and start to accumulate 'junk miles' – a running term that describes time spent training that provides little in the way of results. LSD training is a viable and useful form of training but it is only one weapon in your cardio armoury. Use it but don't abuse it if you want to see your fitness levels climb ever upwards.

Example workout: forty minutes of easy paced running. At the end of such a workout you should feel you have plenty more miles left in the tank.

Tempo training

Where LSD is all about slowness and steadiness, tempo training, also known as Fast Continuous Running (FCR) and Anaerobic Threshold training (AnT) are the opposite. Conducted at eighty-five to ninety per cent of your age-adjusted maximum heart rate, tempo training is about working as hard as you can while still remaining aerobic.

Tempo workouts tend to be considerably shorter than LSD-type training sessions, but that doesn't mean they are easy. A good tempo workout is as much about pushing your mind as it is your muscles, heart and lungs. Work at your maximum sustainable speed – at a rate where, if you went any faster, you would have to slow down. This 'red line' is also known as your anaerobic threshold. This is the point where you are just below the speed at which lactic acid would rise uncontrollably and force you to slow down or stop.

In running and rowing terms, 5,000 m is a good distance to aim for with this type of workout whereas 1,000–1,500 m is a good tempo distance for a competent swimmer. Unless you are an extremely well-trained endurance athlete, a tempo training session should be limited to around twenty to thirty minutes in duration.

Tempo training workouts are best thought of as time trials or races. Because of the intensity of this type of workout you should make sure you are well rested before and plan for adequate recovery after each tempo training session.

Example workout: A 10-mi cycling time trial against the clock. At the end of this workout you should feel you have given it your all and have very little energy left.

Fartlek training

This funny word is Swedish for speed play and describes a variably paced workout where you run/cycle/row etc. at different speeds and for different durations based on how you feel and what you are trying to achieve from your workouts.

The hardest part about Fartlek training is having the motivation to actually get out and do it! If you are feeling a little bit flat or are generally lacking in enthusiasm, it's very easy to turn a planned Fartlek training session into an easy LSD session instead.

Fartlek works best when you have physical markers to use to control the different speeds at which you intend to work at. Park benches, lamp posts, blocks of buildings etc. are all good ways to control your workout. Training with a partner can also work well. Take it in turns to challenge one another, but remember that your aim is not to run the other fellow into the ground, merely have a good workout.

A Fartlek training session should be more demanding than an LSD workout but not as tough as a tempo workout and provides a nice bridge between the two. Remember to include a warm-up and cool-down in your Fartlek sessions and mix both the speed and duration of the efforts in the workout.

Example workout: a thirty-minute Fartlek running workout might look like this...

- Minutes 0–5 – a steady jog progressing to a slightly faster run to warm up
- Minutes 6–8 – fifty fast, long strides alternated with fifty steps of jogging
- Minutes 9–10 – walking to recover
- Minutes 11–15 – sustained 'tempo' speed running
- Minutes 16–19 – jogging to recover
- Minutes 20–25 – repeated hill sprints with a walk-back recovery
- Minutes 26–30 – walk/jog to recover and cool down

Interval training

Alternating periods of intense exercise with periods of rest is called interval training. Interval training is probably the most versatile of all the cardiovascular training methods as, by manipulating the length and difficulty of the work periods, intervals can be used to develop aerobic or anaerobic fitness and can be modified to suit beginner, intermediate or advanced exercisers.

Like most forms of cardiovascular training, intervals can be performed using pretty much all training modalities, from cycling to running and from swimming to skipping. Interval training exposes you to a level of exercise that you are not normally able to sustain for long periods. For example, if you are a rower with a best-ever 5,000-m time of twenty minutes, your average speed is two minutes per 500 m. Rowing further at the same or a slower speed will do little to increase your performance. However, rowing repeated efforts of 1,000 m at one minute and fifty seconds per 500 m will train your body to better deal with a faster pace. Allowing time for the necessary physiological adaptations to occur, you will find your pace over 5,000 m increases.

This reduction in exercise duration might suggest that interval training is not a good training system for weight control. In actuality, the opposite is true. Interval training is an especially effective method for fat-burning despite, somewhat ironically, usually being shorter than tempo, Fartlek or LSD workouts.

Your body runs on the energy it derives from food. Protein, fats and carbohydrates all provide energy, which is commonly measured in calories or kilojoules. Excess food energy is converted and stored as fat that must then be 'burnt off' through exercise and other forms of physical activity.

Working at a higher than normal level of intensity uses more energy in the same way that driving your car faster burns more fuel. Exercising at a lower level of intensity, using LSD-type training, for example, means you use a relatively small amount of energy to fuel your workouts. This is good news if you want to be as economic with your energy as possible but many people actually want the opposite; they want to use lots of energy to facilitate fat loss. Step on the gas and move up and out of your comfort zone! Despite the fact your workouts are likely to be shorter, you'll actually use more energy and, assuming your diet is in balance, this energy will come from your fat stores.

As well as being more 'energy expensive', interval training also elevates your metabolism (the rate at which your body uses energy) for as many as twenty-four hours after the cessation of exercise. This is due to a phenomenon called Excessive Post-exercise Oxygen Consumption (EPOC), and something that used to be called oxygen debt or after-burn.

In simple terms, interval training produces a metabolic waste product called lactic acid. That's the stuff that makes your muscles burn when you are working especially hard. Once you finish your interval-training workout, some lactic acid remains in your system. This has to be flushed out. Your body uses oxygen to do this.

As a result, your heart rate, breathing rate, metabolic rate and therefore energy expenditure remains slightly elevated after an interval-training workout. It's as though you are getting extra interest on your original efforts! EPOC results in a significant additional energy cost per workout compared to typical LSD-type training where no such EPOC occurs.

To summarize: interval-training workouts will increase your fitness, save you time, burn more calories and can be customized to suit your fitness levels and goals. The question is: why wouldn't you do interval training?

Designing an interval-training workout is simple enough; you merely select the work-to-rest ratio suited to your training goal, decide how many repeats you are going to perform (which depends on your current level of fitness) and off you go! Bear in mind that an interval-training session that looks okay on paper is usually much more challenging in reality. Be conservative in your planning if you are new to interval training so you don't bite off more than you can chew. It's better to underestimate your abilities and leave room for improvement than overestimate them and attempt a workout you cannot complete. Here are some guidelines to help you design your own interval-training sessions. Simply adhere to the prescribed work-to-rest ratios and adjust the durations and repetitions according to your current abilities.

- **Aerobic intervals** - work-to-rest intervals: 1:0.5 to 1:1, e.g. fast running for five – minutes, walk/jog for two and a half minutes to five minutes to recover. Repeat three to five times.
- **Lactic acid anaerobic intervals** - work-to-rest intervals 1:3, e.g. hard rowing for one minute, easy rowing for three minutes to recover. Repeat six to eight times.
- **Creatine Phosphate anaerobic intervals (the energy source for flat-out sprinting)** - work-to-rest intervals 1:9, e.g. ten second exercise bike sprint, ninety seconds slow pedalling to recover. Repeat ten to fifteen times.

As you can see, the more intense the effort, the longer the rest period is, proportional to the work period.

Breaking the rules – Tabata interval training

Tabata interval training, the brainchild of Japanese sports scientist Dr Izumi Tabata, breaks all the work-to-rest rules discussed above to create a hellish but supremely effective training protocol that involves as little as four minutes of exercise. Four minutes might sound like a breeze, but the intensity of this type of workout means that four minutes is plenty!

In his studies, Dr Tabata tested his protocol on already-fit Olympic speed skaters and, despite the very brief workouts and the experience of the skaters, it increased their anaerobic and aerobic fitness significantly. This method also creates a significant EPOC, which means that a workout as short as only four minutes can still result in fat loss.

The nuts and bolts of Tabata interval training are simple: work as hard as you can for twenty seconds, rest for ten seconds and then repeat eight to ten times to total four to five minutes of work. Needless to say, you should always warm up for a few minutes before and cool down for a few minutes after so, in reality, this probably equals a workout around fifteen minutes in duration. Nevertheless, Tabata interval training provides an extremely time-efficient, if slightly masochistic, way to obtain and maintain a good level of fitness.

You can apply the Tabata interval training protocol to a wide number of exercise modalities. Sprinting, squat jumps, kettlebell swings, burpees, tyre flips and rowing are just some of the choices available. The main caveat of Tabata interval training is that, whatever exercise you select, you perform each set to your absolute maximum ability. No pacing, no saving yourself for a strong finish – perform as much work as possible in the first twenty seconds and then try to maintain that work rate for the remaining intervals. In reality, you probably won't be able to do this, but that's what you have to strive for. If you are ever short of time and have only got five or ten minutes to squeeze in a training session, you now have an excuse-free training method in Tabata intervals.

Hill training

I was always told that hill training was speed training in disguise and, while that's true, hill training can be a whole lot more than that!

Hill training is a variation of interval training but with the obvious addition of having to overcome gravity as you slog up an incline. Hill training is really only the reserve of runners and cyclists – you can't really row uphill, after all! If, however, running and cycling are not your thing, you can also get a great hill-training workout by strapping on a rucksack or weighted vest and power-walking uphill. In my own experience, I have found steep uphill walking while wearing a weighted vest to provide a tremendous leg and lung workout without the impact associated with running.

There are two main approaches to hill training – short and sharp or long and mean. Short and sharp hills will develop leg power and anaerobic fitness whereas long and mean hills will develop aerobic fitness and leg endurance. The actual length and steepness of the hill you choose should depend on your fitness level, but whether you are trying to sprint up a short, steep incline or conquer the biggest, longest hill in your area, you should aim to make your ascension as fast as possible.

Finding good hills may take some exploring, but once you have located a suitable incline, you have a great training venue. You can combine your hill training with any number of other types of exercise. For example, do ten burpees at the bottom of your hill, run up to the top and then perform twenty alternating lunges. Walk back down to the bottom and repeat.

Alternatively, and if your hill is sufficiently long, break your hill into four equal sections marked with cones or conveniently located markers like park benches or lamp posts. Run up to the first marker and then jog back to the beginning. Run up to the second marker and then back to the start. Repeat this process by running up to the third and finally the forth. Rest for a moment (you'll probably need it!) and then walk back to the bottom and repeat the entire sequence a few more times.

If you can't find a suitable hill, consider making your hill training more urban by running up flights of stairs instead. Sports stadiums, office blocks and apartment blocks are all viable stair-running venues, but please make sure you are not trespassing and ensure that you have permission before embarking on a stair-climbing workout. As before, if you prefer a lower impact but still vertically challenging workout, try walking up flights of stairs while wearing a backpack or weighted vest or carrying weights in your hands instead of running. It's no less effective but potentially more joint-friendly.

You can combine stair climbing with lots of other exercises. For example, perform a set of ten press-ups on each landing or place some weights at the bottom of your stairwell and perform a set of dumb-bell squats, curls and presses between each ascent.

One of my favourite stair-climbing workouts involves nothing more than a willing partner and a suitably long flight of stairs – use a six-storey block of flats or similar. Decide who is going to run the stairs first. This person then designates an exercise for the non-climbing partner to do at the bottom while the climber runs up and then down the stairs. The person at the bottom tries to do as many repetitions in the time it takes the runner to ascend and descend. The roles are then reversed. On completion, and after a quick pause for breath, another exercise is selected and the process repeated. Continue in this alternating fashion for a predetermined length of time, e.g. thirty minutes, or for a set number of exercises, e.g. ten.

As you can see, cardio training can be a whole lot more involved than simply heading out for a jog around the same old route or turning up to some arbitrary exercise class at a local leisure centre. By using a variety of cardio training modalities and methods, keeping your heart and lungs in great shape need never be boring and your fitness levels will climb and climb!

CHAPTER FIVE

Bodyweight and low-tech exercise library

There are, in all likelihood, thousands of bodyweight and low-tech exercises to choose from and many of them will have more than one name. To help get you started, here is a list of exercises that have been 'field tested' for effectiveness. In a nutshell, to make it into this library, the exercise in question had to be a good one that provided plenty of bang for your buck and delivered results while being safe and relatively straightforward to perform.

Feel free to add your own favourite exercises but, remember, in exercise as in life, more complex doesn't necessarily mean more effective. Often, the simplest solution is the best and, while you could be doing one-armed half-twisting reverse press-ups against a wall, the good old press-up will probably get the job done in all but the minority of cases.

Upper-body push

Pressing exercises work your shoulders, chest and triceps, the degree being dictated by the position of your body and hand placement. Of all the bodyweight exercises, press-ups are probably the most well-known. In fact, the humble press-up is, I suspect, the most well-known exercise in the world!

Note – muscles are listed in order of importance in the exercises being described. In the majority of pushing exercises, pectoralis major, deltoids and triceps are working together BUT it is possible to identify the main muscle involved and that is the one listed first.

Press-ups

Targets: pectoralis major, deltoids, triceps

How to perform: squat down and place your hands on the floor, shoulder-width apart. Walk your feet back so your shoulders, hips and feet form a straight line. Keep your abs tight and your neck long. Bend your arms and lower your chest so it lightly touches the floor. Push back up to full arm extension. Do not lead with your head or allow your hips to rise or drop.

Hints, tips and variations: you can make this exercise easier by bending your legs and resting on your knees: the so-called three-quarter press-up. The closer your knees are to your hands, the easier the press-up becomes. If you want a more demanding exercise, elevate your feet. The closer your feet are to shoulder-height (or above) the more demanding the exercise becomes; however, once your feet are higher than shoulder-height, you place more emphasis on your deltoids. You can also increase the range of movement at your shoulders by placing your hands on elevated platforms, such as a couple of house bricks or thick books. While this does make the exercise more demanding, the extra shoulder stress may be problematic for some.

Press-ups – the king of bodyweight upper-body exercises

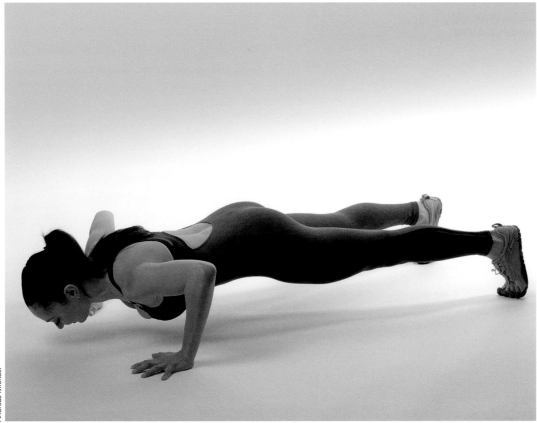

Andreas Michael

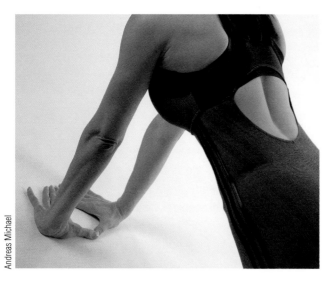

Andreas Michael

Diamond press-ups

Targets: triceps, pectoralis major, deltoids

How to perform: place your hands on the floor so that your first finger and thumb form a diamond shape. Adopt your regular press-up position. Bend your arms and lower your chest to your hands. Push back up to full arm extension and repeat.

Hints, tips and variations: As with all forms of press-up, resting on your knees makes the exercise easier while elevating your feet makes it more challenging. Keep your core tight and do not allow your hips to lift or drop.

Diamond press-ups – tough on the triceps

Staggered hand press-ups

Targets: pectoralis major, deltoids, triceps

How to perform: in the press-up position, place one hand directly beneath your shoulder and one hand below your hip. The hand below your shoulder will be the most heavily loaded while the hand at hip-level is only for assistance. Bend your arms and lower your chest to the floor and press back up. On completion of a set, rest a moment and swap arms.

Hints, tips and variations: this exercise is a good transition movement if you want to progress to one-armed press-ups. Use your lower arm less and less until you are able to lift and lower yourself using one arm only.

Staggered hand press-ups – a stepping stone to one-armed press-ups

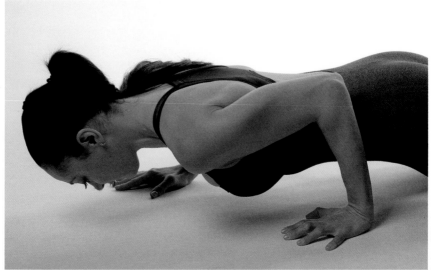

Andreas Michael

No Gym? No problem!

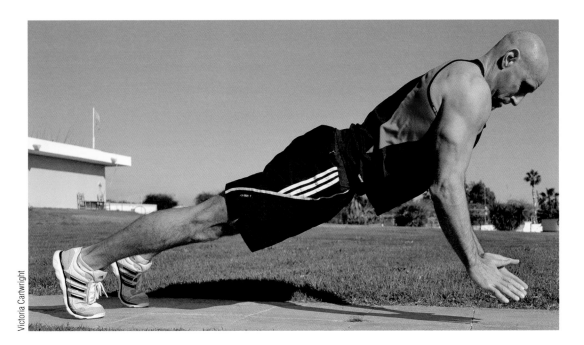

Victoria Cartwright

Plyometric press-ups

Targets: pectoralis major, deltoids, triceps

How to perform: with your hands shoulder-width apart, bend your arms and lower your chest to lightly touch the floor. Extend your arms explosively and push yourself off the ground. Land on slightly bent elbows and then repeat.

Hints, tips and variations: if you like, add a clap while you are in mid-air. If you have a history of wrist problems, this exercise should be performed with caution, if at all.

Plyometric press-ups
– getting some air!

Pike press-ups work
your shoulders hard

Pike press-ups

Targets: deltoids, triceps, pectoralis major

How to perform: adopt the press-up position with your arms straight and core tight. Push your body backwards and lift your hips so that your body resembles an inverted V shape. Bend your arms and lower your head towards the floor and then press back up.

Hints, tips and variations: you can make this exercise more demanding by elevating your feet. This is a good alternative to handstand press-ups (see page 90).

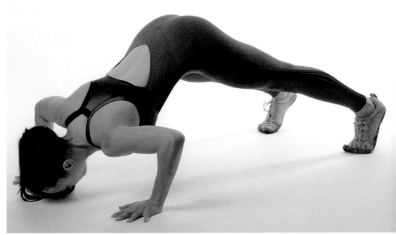

Andreas Michael

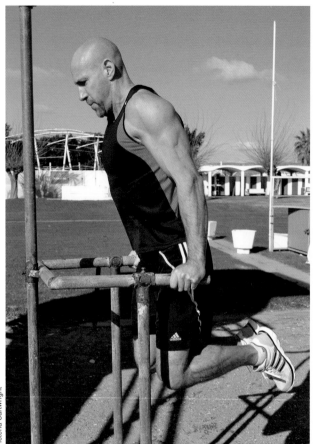

Victoria Cartwright

Dips

Targets: triceps, pectoralis major, deltoids

Equipment: dipping bars, chairs, a step or an exercise bench

How to perform: using a dip station, support your weight on extended arms. Bend your legs and cross your ankles. Keeping your chest up, bend your arms and descend until your elbows are bent just beyond ninety degrees. Push back up and repeat.

Hints, tips and variations: make dips more demanding by tying a weight around your waist or wearing a weighted vest or backpack. This exercise can also be performed on an exercise bench, at the bottom of a flight of stairs or between two sturdy chairs.

Dips – an advanced arm, chest and shoulder exercise

Isometric chest press

Targets: pectoralis major, deltoids, triceps

How to perform: standing or seated, place your hands in front of your chest in a 'prayer' position. Push your hands together as hard as you can for ten to fifteen seconds and then release.

Hints, tips and variations: avoid holding your breath as this can adversely affect your blood pressure.

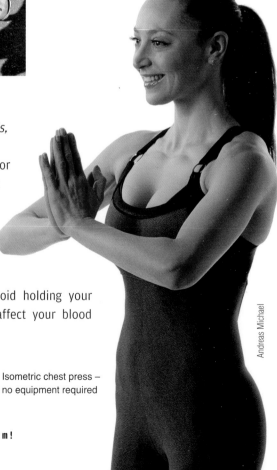

Andreas Michael

Isometric chest press – no equipment required

Dumb-bell curl and press

Targets: deltoids, biceps, triceps

Equipment: dumb-bells, a barbell, sandbag(s) or a resistance band

How to perform: stand with a dumb-bell in each hand and your feet hip-width apart. Bend your arms and raise the dumb-bells to shoulder-height and then press them directly overhead. Lower the weights back to your shoulders and then back down to your sides.

Hints, tips and variations: perform this exercise with both arms simultaneously or using an alternating arm action as preferred. Keep your chest up and your body rigid throughout; no swinging with your back or jerking with your legs. This exercise can also be performed two-handed using a barbell, sandbag or resistance band.

Two exercises in one make the dumb-bell curl and press a very efficient exercise

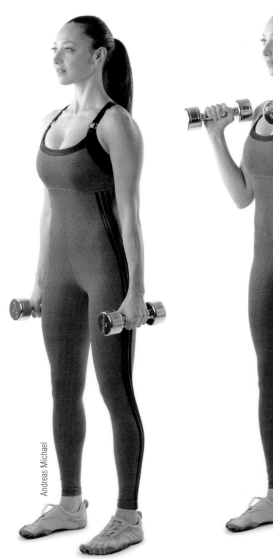

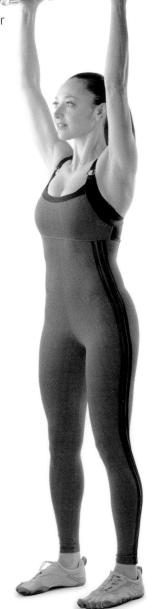

Andreas Michael

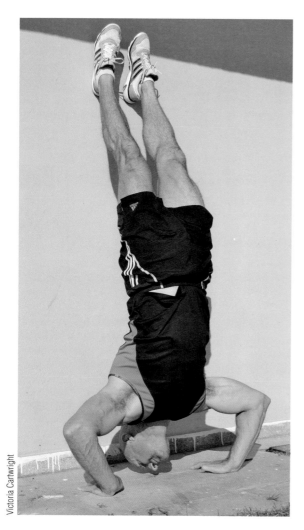

Victoria Cartwright

Handstand press-ups

Targets: deltoids, triceps

How to perform: squat down and place your hands shoulder-width apart around 6 in/15 cm from a flat and sturdy wall. Kick up and into a handstand position with your legs resting against the wall for support. Bend your arms and lower your head down to lightly touch the floor. Push back up and repeat.

Hints, tips and variations: this is a tough exercise! If, initially, handstand press-ups are too demanding you can perform pike press-ups (see page 87). Also consider placing a rolled towel, cushion or exercise mat under your head in case you should inadvertently descend too quickly.

One-and-a-half side lateral raises

Targets: deltoids

How to perform: when either standing or seated, raise your arms straight up and out to the side to shoulder-level. Lower your arms halfway and then lift them back up again. Lower them all the way down to your side and then repeat.

Hints, tips and variations: this exercise is best suited to moderate to high repetitions. Expect this exercise to make your deltoids burn!

Handstand press-ups build real pushing strength

No weights required but still an effective exercise

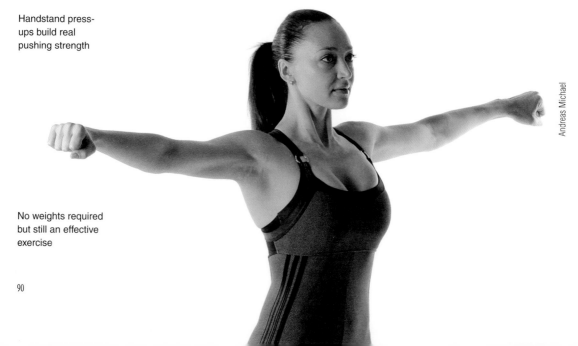

Andreas Michael

Resistance band lateral raises

Targets: deltoids

Equipment: resistance band

How to perform: stand on the middle of your resistance band and hold an end in each hand. With a slight bend in your elbows, lift your hands up and out to shoulder-height. Lower your arms and repeat.

Hints, tips and variations: if your band is short or especially strong, perform this exercise one arm at a time and stand so that there is more slack available.

Shoulder presses

Targets: deltoids, triceps

Equipment: barbell, dumb-bells, kettlebells, a sandbag, a resistance band or a rock

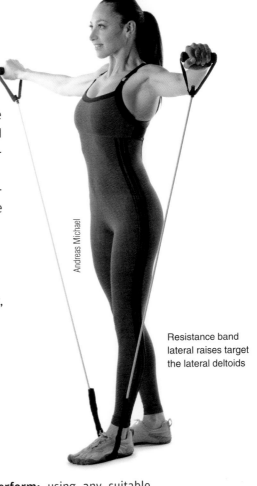

Andreas Michael

Resistance band lateral raises target the lateral deltoids

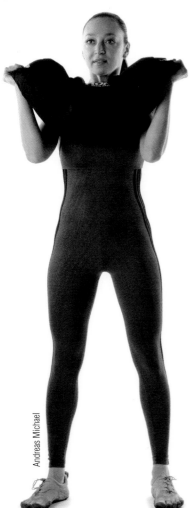

Andreas Michael

How to perform: using any suitable object – kettlebell, dumb-bell, rock, sandbag, etc. – stand with the weight racked at shoulder-height with your forearms as close to vertical as possible. Keeping your knees slightly bent and your core braced, push the object up and overhead to arm's length. Lower to the starting position and repeat.

Hints, tips and variations: if using dumb-bells or single weights, you can perform this exercise one arm at a time or using both arms together. The single-arm version of this exercise places an additional load on your core muscles.

Simply take a heavy object and press up from your shoulders to above your head!

Upper-body pull

It's very important that, for every pushing exercise you perform, you do a pulling exercise. This ensures that your muscles, which are generally arranged in pairs, are equally developed on the front AND the rear of your body. This will create a more aesthetically pleasing physique and also ensures that your joints are structurally balanced from front to rear. Unbalanced pairs of muscles are more prone to injury as they can adversely affect the alignment of your joints and increase your risk of joint dysfunction.

Note – muscles are listed in order of importance in the exercise being described. In the majority of pulling exercises, latissimus dorsi, middle trapezius, rhomboids, posterior deltoids and biceps are working together BUT it is possible to identify the main muscle involved and that is the one listed first.

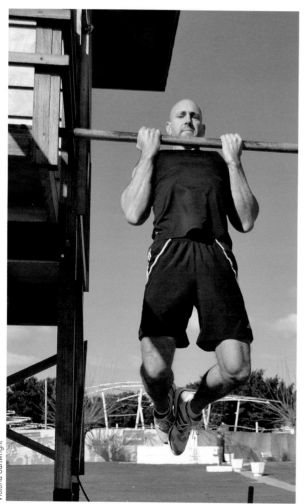

Victoria Cartwright

Chin-ups

Targets: latissimus dorsi, biceps

Equipment: chin-up bar or tree branch

How to perform: grasp a suitable overhead bar, beam or branch with an underhand, slightly narrower than shoulder-width grip and hang at full stretch. Bend your arms and, leading down and back with your elbows, pull yourself up until your chin is above the level of the bar. Slowly lower yourself down to full stretch and repeat.

Hints, tips and variations: make this exercise more demanding by tying a weight around your waist or wearing a weighted vest or a backpack. Make this exercise easier by placing a sturdy chair behind you and using your legs for assistance.

Chin-ups use an underhand grip

No Gym? No problem!

Pull-ups

Targets: latissimus dorsi, biceps

Equipment: chin-up bar or tree branch

How to perform: grasp a suitable overhead bar, beam or branch with an overhand, slightly wider than shoulder-width grip and hang at full stretch. Bend your arms and, leading down and back with your elbows, pull yourself up until your chin is above the level of the bar. Slowly lower yourself down to full stretch and repeat.

Hints, tips and variations: make this exercise more demanding by tying a weight around your waist or wearing a weighted vest or a backpack. Make this exercise easier by placing a sturdy chair behind you and using your legs for assistance.

Climber pull-ups

Targets: latissimus dorsi, biceps

Equipment: chin-up bar or tree branch

How to perform: using an overhand and slightly wider than shoulder-width grip, bend your arms and pull yourself up and over so your chin touches your left hand. Keeping your arms bent, traverse along the bar so that your chin touches your right hand. Extend your arms and return to the starting position. Repeat but start by pulling yourself up and over to the opposite side. Continue alternating sides for the duration of your set.

Hints, tips and variations: make this exercise more demanding by tying a weight around your waist or wearing a weighted vest or a backpack. Make this exercise easier by placing a sturdy chair behind you and using your legs for assistance.

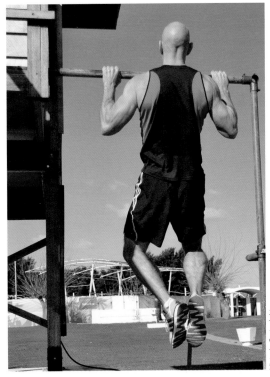

Pull-ups use an overhand grip

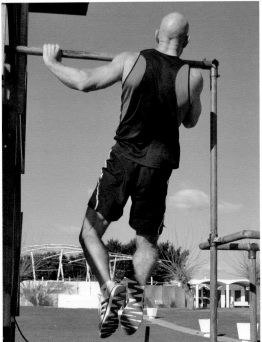

Climber pull-ups feature a challenging side-to-side movement

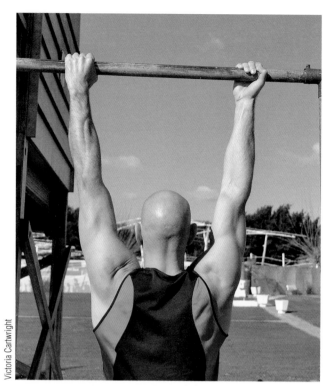

Mixing it up with mixed-grip pull-ups

Mixed-grip pull-ups

Targets: latissimus dorsi, biceps

Equipment: chin-up bar or tree branch

How to perform: perform pull-ups in the usual fashion but with one palm turned away from and one palm facing you. Swap hands on a set-by-set basis.

Hints, tips and variations: make this exercise more demanding by tying a weight around your waist or wearing a weighted vest or a backpack. Make this exercise easier by placing a sturdy chair behind you and using your legs for assistance.

Towel pull-ups

Targets: latissimus dorsi, biceps, forearms

Equipment: chin-up bar or tree branch and towel

How to perform: hang two towels over your pull-up bar and grab an end in each hand. Grip the towels very tightly! Hang at full stretch and then perform your pull-ups in the usual fashion. Because your hands will be below the level of the pull-up bar, pull up until your hands touch your shoulders.

Hints, tips and variations: make this exercise more demanding by tying a weight around your waist or wearing a weighted vest or a backpack. Make this exercise easier by placing a sturdy chair behind you and using your legs for assistance.

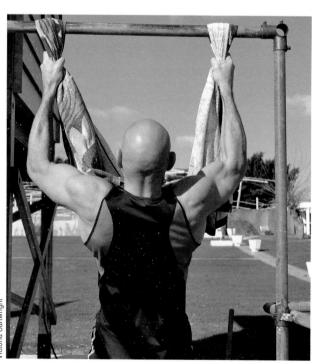

Towel pull-ups
develop an iron grip!

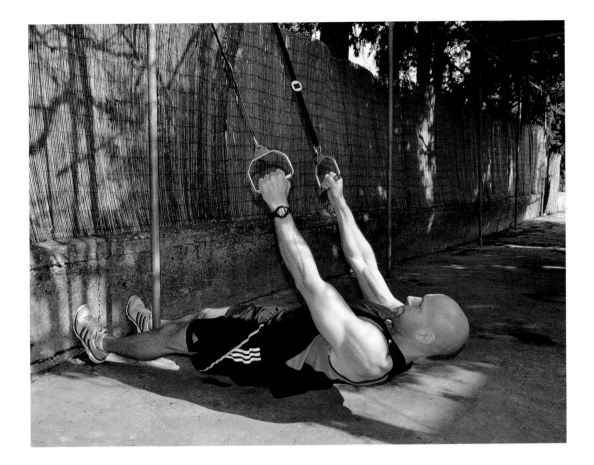

Body rows

Targets: latissimus dorsi, middle trapezius, rhomboids, posterior deltoids, biceps

Equipment: suspension trainer, Smith machine or squat rack and barbell

How to perform: sit below a waist-high suspension trainer, a sturdy bar such as a barbell placed in a squat rack, a Smith machine or a heavy, stable table; a strong broom resting between two chair backs can also work. Grasp the bar with an overhand shoulder-width grip. Extend your legs so your body and arms are straight and your weight is supported on your heels and by your hands only. Bend your arms and pull yourself up so your chest touches the bar. Try to lead with your elbows and keep your wrists straight. Extend your arms and then repeat.

Hints, tips and variations: Keep your body absolutely straight during this exercise. To make the exercise less demanding, raise the level of the bar or the suspension-trainer handles to place more weight on your feet. To make the exercise more challenging, elevate your feet, rest a weight across your hips or wear a weighted vest.

Body rows – a great back builder

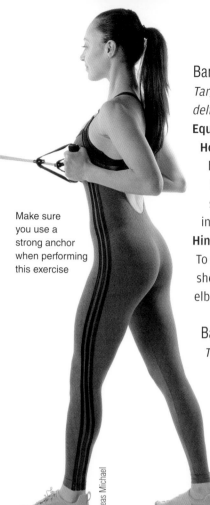

Make sure you use a strong anchor when performing this exercise

Andreas Michael

Band rows

Targets: latissimus dorsi, middle trapezius, rhomboids, posterior deltoids, biceps

Equipment: resistance band

How to perform: anchor the centre of your band securely at waist-height. Grasp the ends and step back until your arms are straight in front of you and the band is sufficiently tensioned. With your knees slightly bent for stability, lead with your elbows and pull your hands into your lower ribs. Slowly extend your arms and repeat.

Hints, tips and variations: this exercise can also be performed seated. To emphasize your upper back, specifically the muscles between your shoulder blades, pull your hands up to chest-height and keep your elbows level with your shoulders.

Band pull-aparts

Targets: middle trapezius, posterior deltoids

Equipment: resistance band

How to perform: hold a resistance band in both hands and at chest-height. Extend your arms out in front of you. Keeping your arms slightly bent but rigid, spread your arms and stretch the bend out and across your chest. Pause for a second before slowly returning to the starting position and repeating.

Hints, tips and variations: keep your chest up and knees slightly bent at all times. This exercise can also be performed with an old-fashioned chest expander.

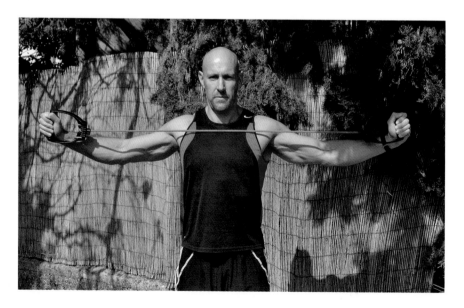

Band pull-aparts – dig out that old chest expander!

No Gym? No problem!

Isometric towel shrugs

Targets: upper trapezius

Equipment: towel

How to perform: stand on the middle of a long towel and grab an end in each hand. With your hands by your sides, shrug your shoulders upwards while gripping the towel as hard as you can to prevent movement. Shrug down as hard as you can and then release.

Hints, tips and variations: avoid holding your breath as this can adversely affect your blood pressure. If you are using a short towel, instead of standing on the towel simply kneel on it.

Isometric towel row

Targets: latissimus dorsi, middle trapezius, rhomboids, biceps

Equipment: towel

How to perform: stand in the middle of a long towel and grab an end in each hand. Bend your knees slightly and then hinge forwards from your hips so your upper body is inclined to around eighty degrees. Lift your chest and arch your lower back. Position your hands on the towel so that your elbows are bent. Without moving your upper body and while gripping the towel as tightly as you can, pull as hard as possible as though you were performing a bent-over row.

Hints, tips and variations: avoid holding your breath as this can adversely affect your blood pressure.

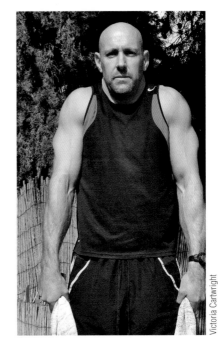

Victoria Cartwright

Shrugs build the upper traps and shoulders

Pull as hard as you can!

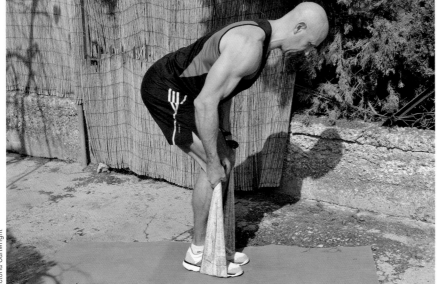

Victoria Cartwright

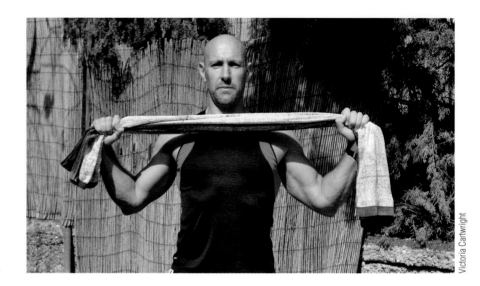

Towel pull-downs –
simple but effective

Towel pull-downs

Targets: latissimus dorsi, middle trapezius, rhomboids, biceps

Equipment: towel

How to perform: stand and hold a towel with a slightly wider than shoulder-width grip. Raise the towel above your head. Pull the ends of the towel apart as you pull down to touch the front of your neck. Keep pulling the ends apart. Raise your arms up above your head and repeat.

Hints, tips and variations: if limited shoulder flexibility makes this exercise uncomfortable, move your hands further apart. Do not be tempted to pull the towel down behind your neck as this can lead to injury.

Eccentric pull-up/chin-up (not pictured)

Targets: latissimus dorsi, biceps

Equipment: chin-up bar or tree branch

How to perform: using a step, get into the upper position of a pull-up (hands facing away from you) or a chin-up (hands facing towards you). Shift your weight onto your arms and cross your feet behind you. Slowly lower yourself down to full arm extension and then, using your legs, return to the starting position and repeat. Continue until you are no longer able to control your descent.

Hints, tips and variations: eccentric pull-ups/chin-ups are a great way to perform these exercises if you are unable to execute the regular version. Even if you can't pull yourself up, you can probably lower yourself down as you are stronger eccentrically than you are concentrically. Perform pull-ups/chin-ups while wearing a weighted vest, backpack or weight around your waist and you will expose your muscles to greater load than if you were doing standard reps. Be aware, eccentric training can cause SEVERE muscle soreness!

Lower body

Leg training can be exhausting. Those big thigh and hip muscles use a lot of energy and this usually correlates with high heart and breathing rates and some weakness at the knees if you are working especially hard. Subsequently, some exercisers pay less attention than they ought to to their leg training or, in some cases, don't do any specific leg exercises at all. While running and cycling will help to keep your legs in shape, for total development, muscular balance and optimal function you must train your legs!

Note – muscles are listed in order of importance in the exercise being described. In the majority of lower-body exercises, quadriceps, hamstrings and gluteus maximus are working together BUT it is possible to identify the main muscle involved and that is the one listed first.

Squats

Targets: quadriceps, hamstrings, gluteus maximus

How to perform: stand with your feet shoulder-width apart and your toes turned slightly outwards. With your chest up and head facing directly forwards, push your hips back, bend your knees and squat down until your thighs are parallel to the floor or slightly lower. Stand back up and repeat.

Hints, tips and variations: don't do shallow squats – they may be easier on your leg muscles but they are actually harder on your knees as you stop at a mechanically disadvantageous position. No need to go to full knee flexion either where, again, you might injure your knees. Slightly below parallel (ninety degrees of knee flexion) is about right. Do not allow your lower back to become rounded at the bottom of a squat.

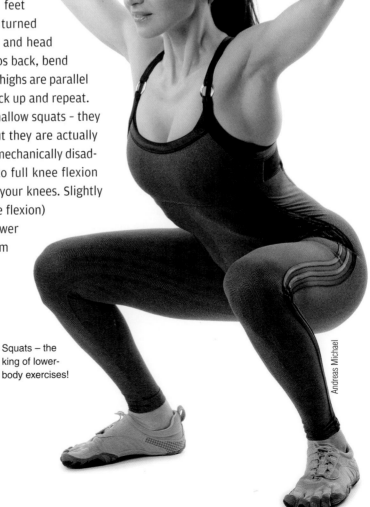

Squats – the king of lower-body exercises!

Andreas Michael

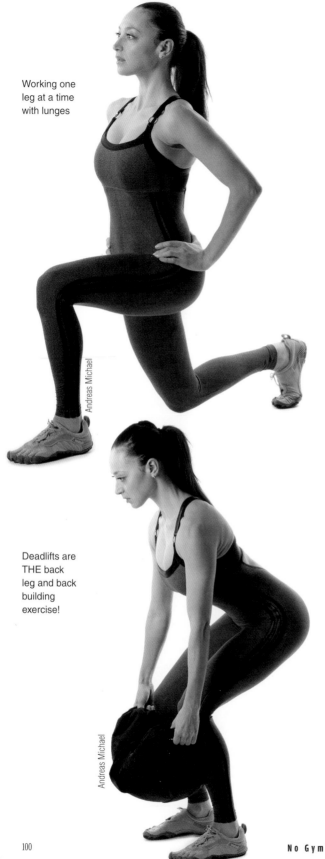

Working one leg at a time with lunges

Andreas Michael

Deadlifts are THE back leg and back building exercise!

Andreas Michael

Lunges

Targets: quadriceps, hamstrings, gluteus maximus

How to perform: stand with your feet together and your hands by your sides. Take a large step forwards and bend your legs. Lower your rear knee to within an inch/a few centimetres of the floor. Your front shin should be vertical and both knees bent to around ninety degrees. Push off your front leg and return to the starting position. Perform another repetition, leading with your opposite leg. Continue alternating legs for the duration of your set.

Hints, tips and variations: lunging on or off a 10-15 cm platform will increase the range of movement of this exercise and make it more demanding. You can also perform backwards lunges, lateral (sideways) lunges and walking lunges for variation.

Deadlifts

Targets: hamstrings, gluteus maximus

Equipment: barbell, dumb-bells, kettle-bells, a sandbag, a heavy rock or a tyre

How to perform: with your weight at your feet, bend your knees, push your hips back and bend forwards. Grasp the weight with a shoulder-width grip. Keeping your chest up and arms straight, stand fully upright. Push your hips to the rear, bend your knees and place the weight back on the floor. Do not allow your lower back to become rounded.

Hints, tips and variations: this exercise can be performed using almost any sufficiently heavy object including a barbell, dumb-bells, a sandbag, a heavy rock or a tyre.

Wrestler squats

Targets: quadriceps, hamstrings, gluteus maximus

Equipment: exercise mat

How to perform: kneel down so that your thighs are vertical, your body is upright and your knees are bent to ninety degrees. From this position step your left leg forwards and plant your foot firmly on the floor in front of you. Next, step through with your right foot and do the same. You should now be in the bottom position of a squat. Without standing up, step back and kneel down with one leg and then the other. Perform your next repetition leading with the opposite leg. Continue alternating legs for the duration of your set.

Hints, tips and variations: perform this exercise on a mat to reduce wear and tear on your knees.

Step-ups

Targets: quadriceps, hamstrings, gluteus maximus

Equipment: step-up bench or box

How to perform: stand facing a sturdy knee-high bench, step or box. Step up onto and then down off the step, making sure your whole foot is on the stepping surface. Try to emphasize your leading leg as much as possible by not pushing off the floor too much. This should feel more like a single-leg squat then climbing a flight of stairs.

Hints, tips and variations: the higher the step, the more demanding this exercise becomes. Add resistance by wearing a backpack or weighted vest or holding weights in your hands, as pictured. Rather than facing towards your step, you can stand sideways on and perform lateral step-ups.

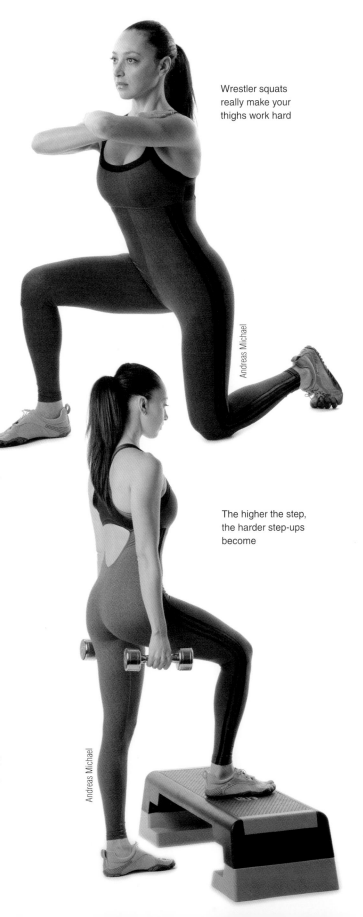

Wrestler squats really make your thighs work hard

The higher the step, the harder step-ups become

Andreas Michael

Andreas Michael

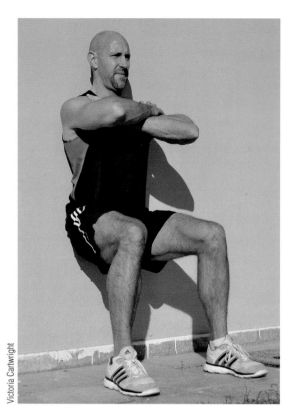

Victoria Cartwright

Isometric wall squats

Targets: quadriceps, hamstrings, gluteus maximus

Equipment: smooth wall

How to perform: stand with your back to a smooth and sturdy wall. With your feet around 18 in/45 cm from the wall, bend your legs and slide down until your thighs are parallel to the floor. Using your legs, push your back against the wall as hard as possible – don't just sit there waiting to get tired!

Hints, tips and variations: avoid holding your breath as this can adversely affect your blood pressure.

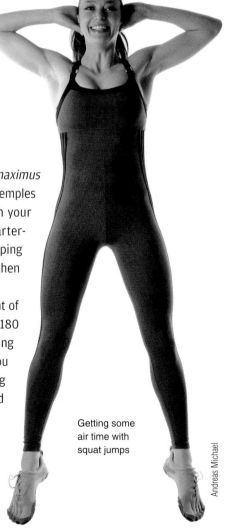

Don't just sit there – try and push the wall down!

Squat jumps

Targets: quadriceps, hamstrings, gluteus maximus

How to perform: with your hands by your temples and your feet shoulder-width apart, push your hips backwards and descend into a quarter-depth squat. Leap up and into the air, jumping as high as you can. Land on bent legs and then immediately perform another repetition.

Hints, tips and variations: add an element of coordination and agility by adding a 180 degree turn to each jump. Alternate turning clockwise and anti-clockwise rep by rep. You can also use your arms when performing this exercise to increase momentum and therefore jumping height.

Getting some air time with squat jumps

Andreas Michael

N o G y m ? N o p r o b l e m !

Jumping lunges

Targets: quadriceps, hamstrings, gluteus maximus

How to perform: take a large step forwards and bend your legs so you are in the bottom position of a lunge. Jump into the air and, while in mid-flight, swap your legs so your rearmost leg is now forwards and vice versa. Land on bent legs, descend and repeat.

Hints, tips and variations: to increase the difficulty of the exercise, add a rotational movement and turn your upper body towards your leading leg. This is a great exercise for tennis players, rugby players and to complement any other sport involving rapid changes in direction.

Rear Foot Elevated Split Squats (RFESS)

Targets: quadriceps, hamstrings, gluteus maximus

Equipment: exercise bench or step

How to Perform: stand with your back to a knee-high bench or step. Place one foot on the bench behind you. Hop forwards and into an extended stance. Bend your legs and lower your rearmost knee to within an inch of the floor. Stand back up and repeat. Swap legs at the end of each set.

Hints, tips and variations: keep your torso upright to maximize the effectiveness of this exercise. If balancing proves difficult, perform this exercise with a chair or similarly sturdy object next to you for added stability.

Andreas Michael

The higher the jump, the harder the workout!

A cumbersome name but this is an effective leg and balance exercise

Andreas Michael

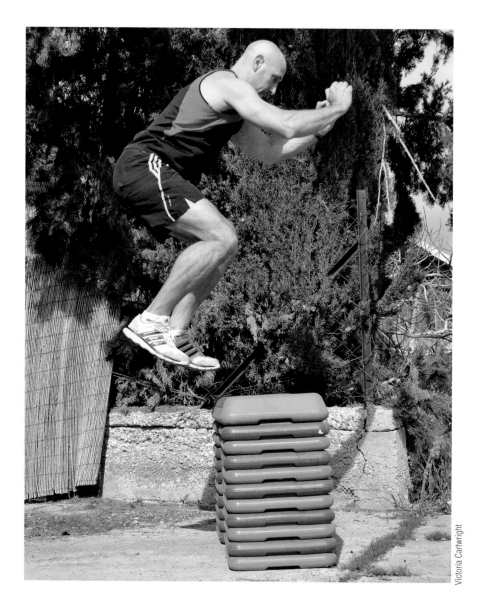

Box jumps will increase leg and lung power

Victoria Cartwright

Box jumps

Targets: quadriceps, hamstrings, gluteus maximus

Equipment: box or step

How to perform: stand around 12 in/30 cm away from a sturdy box or platform. The top of the platform should be roughly level with your knees although a higher platform can also be used. With your feet shoulder-width apart, bend your knees, swing your arms and jump up and onto the box. Land on slightly bent knees. Step back down and repeat.

Hints, tips and variations: alternate the leg with which you step down to ensure you work both legs evenly. Ensure your box is stable and will not tip over easily.

No Gym? No problem!

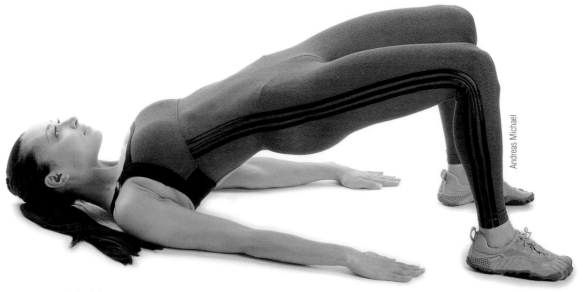

Andreas Michael

Supine hip bridges

Targets: hamstrings, gluteus maximus

Equipment: exercise mat

How to perform: lie on your back with your legs bent and feet flat on the floor as close to your bottom as possible. Place your hands on the floor next to your hips. Push your feet down into the floor and lift your hips upwards. At the top of the movement your knees, hips and shoulders should form a straight line. Lower your bottom back to the floor and repeat.

Hints, tips and variations: place your feet on a 15–30-cm block to increase the range of movement and therefore the difficulty of this exercise. Supine hip bridges can also be performed using one leg at a time – creating a much more demanding hamstring and glute exercise.

Supine hip bridges are a great butt-builder

One-legged Romanian deadlifts

Targets: hamstrings, gluteus maximus

Equipment: dumb-bell or kettlebell (optional)

How to perform: stand with your feet together and your hands by your sides. Shift your weight over onto your left leg. Bend your left knee slightly. Keeping your right leg straight, hinge forwards from the hips until your upper body and trailing leg are roughly parallel to the ground. Stand back up and repeat. On completion of the prescribed number of repetitions, rest a moment and then perform an identical number of repetitions on the opposite leg.

Hints, tips and variations: if balancing proves difficult, perform this exercise with a chair or similarly sturdy object next to you for added stability. As pictured, this exercise can also be performed while holding a weight.

A great hamstring and bottom exercise

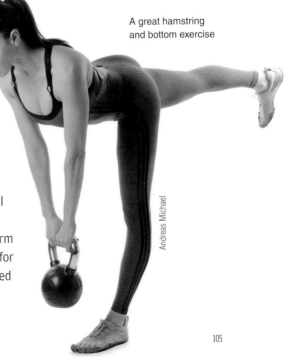

Andreas Michael

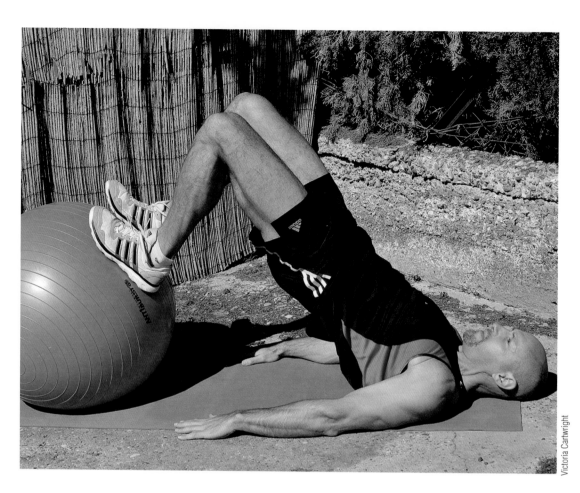

Victoria Cartwright

The SHELC is a total hamstring exercise

Supine Hip Elevation/Leg Curl (SHELC)

Targets: hamstrings, gluteus maximus, erector spinae

Equipment: stability ball

How to perform: lie on your back with your legs straight and your heels resting on the crown of the ball. Place your hands on the floor by your sides for balance. Lift your hips off the floor and then bend your legs, pulling your feet (and the ball) in towards your bottom. Keep pushing your hips up. Slowly extend your legs and lower your hips back down to the floor.

Hints, tips and variations: this exercise can also be performed one leg at a time.

Core

The core is the collective term commonly used to describe the muscles of your midsection. These muscles hold your spine rigid when they contract isometrically, create spinal stability and initiate movements such as bending and twisting. Try to select a variety of core exercises so that you perform movements in a variety of directions. While the rectus abdominus (at the front of your abdomen) is the most commonly used muscle in most core training, it's also important, for spinal health as well as midsection aesthetics, to work the muscles on the side and rear of your core.

Note – muscles are listed in order of importance in the exercise being described. In the majority of core exercises, rectus abdominus, obliques, erector spinae and transverse abdominus are working together BUT it is possible to identify the main muscle involved and that is the one listed first.

Planks

Targets: rectus abdominus, transverse abdominus

Equipment: exercise mat

How to perform: lie on your front with your elbows resting on the floor and your forearms extended in front of you. Lift your hips off the floor so your weight is supported on your arms and feet only. Your shoulders, hips and feet should form a straight line. Without letting your hips lift or drop, hold this position by bracing your abs as hard as you can. Do not hold your breath!

Hints, tips and variations: make this exercise more demanding by lifting one foot off the floor or resting your arms on a medium-sized stability ball.

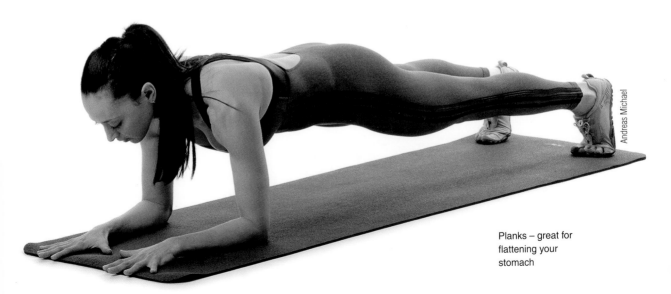

Andreas Michael

Planks – great for flattening your stomach

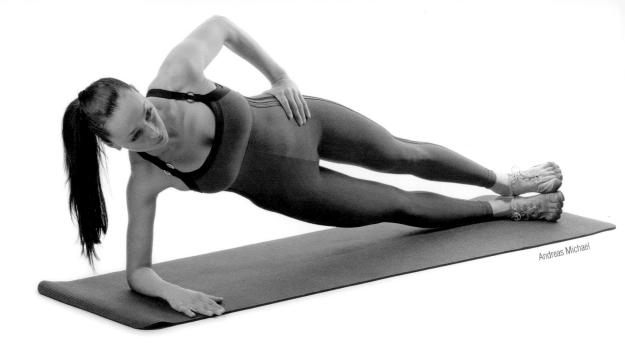

Andreas Michael

Trim your waist with side planks

Side planks

Targets: rectus abdominus, obliques, erector spinae, transverse abdominus

Equipment: exercise mat

How to perform: lie on your side and rest on your elbow. With your body and legs straight, lift your hips off the floor so there is a straight line down the centre of your body. Hold this position for the prescribed duration and then change sides. Do not hold your breath!

Hints, tips and variations: make this exercise more demanding by lifting your upper-most leg to around forty-five degrees.

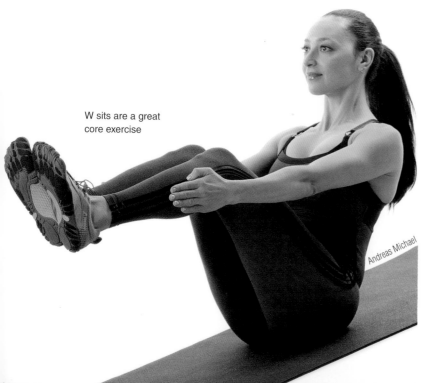

W sits are a great core exercise

Andreas Michael

W sits

Targets: rectus abdominus

Equipment: exercise mat

How to perform: lie on your back with your legs straight and arms above your head. Raise your arms, lift and bend your legs and reach forwards. At the top of this movement you should be balancing on your bottom and lower back. Return to the starting position and repeat.

Hints, tips and variations: for a harder workout, keep your legs straight and reach for your toes; this is called a V sit.

Crunches

Targets: rectus abdominus

Equipment: exercise mat

How to perform: lie on your back with your legs bent so that your thighs are perpendicular to the floor and your knees are bent to ninety degrees. With your hands on your temples, raise your shoulders off the ground as you simultaneously exhale. Hold this contracted position for one to two seconds and then lower your shoulders back to the floor.

Hints, tips and variations: placing your hands across your chest or on the floor next to your hips makes this exercise easier whereas extending your arms above your head makes it more demanding. You can also perform crunches lying across a stability ball, which increases the difficulty significantly.

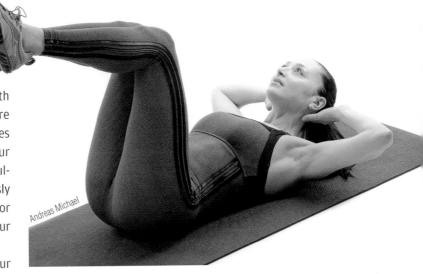

Simple but effective – crunches work

Chinnies

Targets: rectus abdominus, obliques

Equipment: exercise mat

How to perform: lie on your back with your legs straight and your hands on your temples. Sit up and simultaneously bend one leg. Twist your upper body so that your knee lightly touches your opposite elbow. Return to the starting position and then perform another repetition on the opposite side. Continue alternating for the duration of your set.

Hints, tips and variations: to make this exercise more demanding, keep your feet off the ground the whole time. This variation is commonly called a bicycle crunch because of the cycling leg motion.

Chinnies – an exercise borrowed from the world of athletics

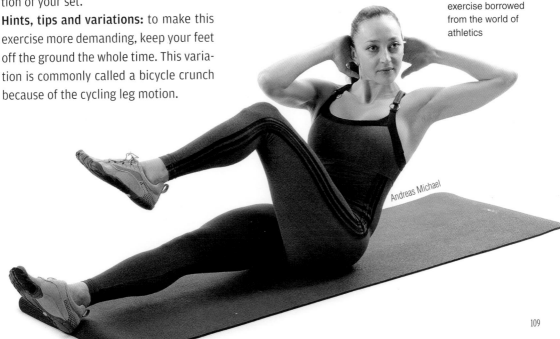

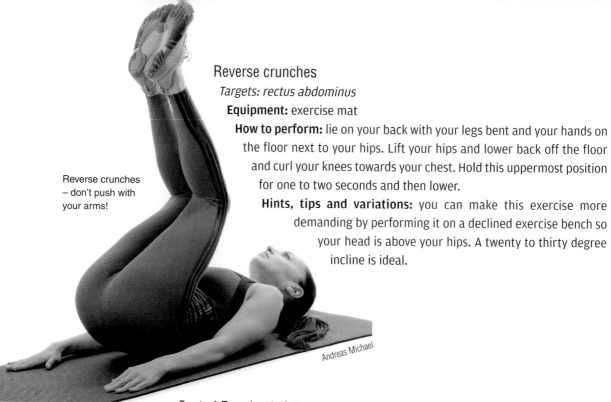

Reverse crunches

Targets: rectus abdominus

Equipment: exercise mat

How to perform: lie on your back with your legs bent and your hands on the floor next to your hips. Lift your hips and lower back off the floor and curl your knees towards your chest. Hold this uppermost position for one to two seconds and then lower.

Hints, tips and variations: you can make this exercise more demanding by performing it on a declined exercise bench so your head is above your hips. A twenty to thirty degree incline is ideal.

Reverse crunches – don't push with your arms!

Andreas Michael

Seated Russian twists

Targets: rectus abdominus, obliques

Equipment: exercise mat; dumb-bell, medicine ball, kettlebell (optional)

How to perform: sit on the floor with your legs bent and feet flat. Sit back so that your upper body is inclined to around forty-five degrees to the floor. Extend your arms perpendicular to your body and clasp your hands together. Without sitting up or back, rotate your upper body to the left and then to the right. Try to turn as far as you can. Perform an equal number of repetitions on each side. Do not hold your breath.

Hints, tips and variations: As pictured, you can make this exercise more demanding by holding a weight in your extended hands.

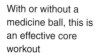

With or without a medicine ball, this is an effective core workout

Andreas Michael

Band twists

Targets: rectus abdominus, obliques

Equipment: resistance band

How to perform: anchor the end of your band securely at shoulder-height and hold the other end in both hands. Standing sideways-on to your anchor, step away to tense the band. Bend your knees slightly and stand with your feet shoulder-width apart for stability. Keeping your arms straight, rotate your upper body 180 degrees away from the anchor. Slowly return to the starting position and repeat. Perform the same number of repetitions on the opposite side.

Hints, tips and variations: this exercise can also be performed using a tornado ball or a medicine ball in a strong bag. Stand with your back to a suitable, strong wall and hold the handle of your bag/ball firmly in both hands. Turn rapidly to your left and right and hit the wall to your sides at around shoulder-level. The momentum of the ball will begin to pull you off balance; don't let it. Keep your core braced at all times.

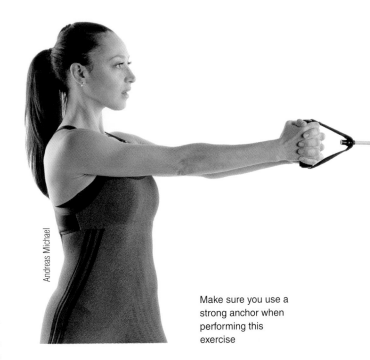

Andreas Michael

Make sure you use a strong anchor when performing this exercise

Boat pose

Targets: rectus abdominus

Equipment: exercise mat

How to perform: sit on the floor with your legs bent and feet close to your bottom. Sit back so your upper body is inclined to around forty-five degrees. Extend your arms so that they are roughly parallel to the floor. Keeping your upper body still, extend your legs so that you are balancing on your bottom and lower back and your body resembles a V shape. Hold this position for as long as possible and then relax.

Hints, tips and variations: the more extended your legs are, the more demanding this exercise becomes. If you are unable to fully extend your knees, bend your legs and perform a static W sit instead (see page 108).

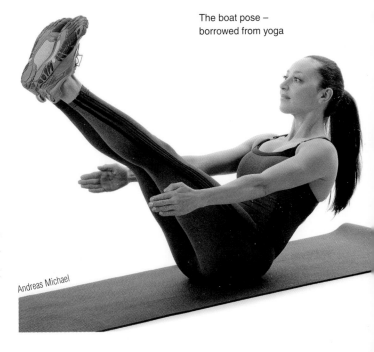

The boat pose – borrowed from yoga

Andreas Michael

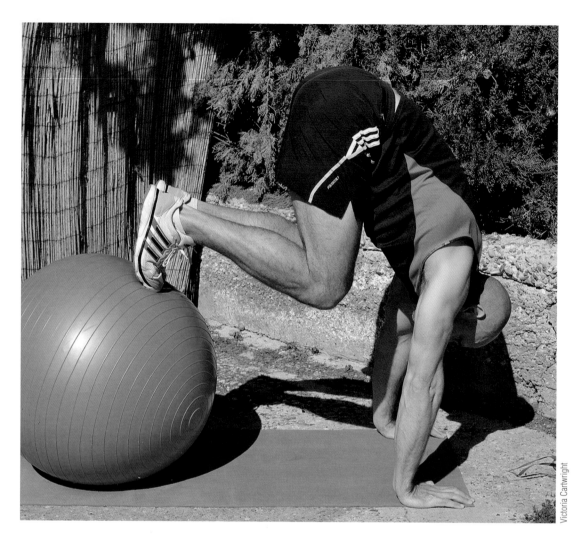

Victoria Cartwright

An effective core, shoulder, arm and balance exercise

Stability ball tucks

Targets: rectus abdominus, hip flexors

Equipment: stability ball

How to perform: place your hands on the floor and your feet on a stability ball - a press-up position with your feet elevated. Using your abdominal muscles, flex and lift your hips and bend your knees so the ball rolls towards your hands. Slowly return to the starting position and repeat.

Hints, tips and variations: this exercise can also be performed using a suspension-training device. Simply put your feet in the end loops instead of resting them on a stability ball.

Stability ball back extensions

Targets: erector spinae

Equipment: stability ball

How to perform: lie face down on a stability ball with your feet against a wall for balance and the ball positioned under your hips. Roll yourself onto the ball and then lift your upper body up and off the ball. Slowly return to the starting position and repeat.

Hints, tips and variations: place your hands behind your back for an easy workout or at your temples for a more demanding one.

Sky divers

Targets: erector spinae

Equipment: exercise mat

How to perform: lie on your front with your legs straight and your hands lightly touching your temples. Squeeze your elbows back. Keeping your feet pressed firmly into the ground, lift your arms, chest, head and shoulders off the floor. Hold this position for the desired duration and then relax.

Hints, tips and variations: this exercise can be performed as a timed isometric hold or for reps. For a more demanding workout, extend your arms away from you to lengthen the lever. To make the exercise less demanding, place your hands behind your lower back.

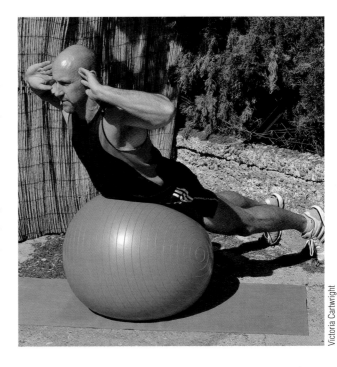

Victoria Cartwright

Stability ball back extensions – a great lower back exercise

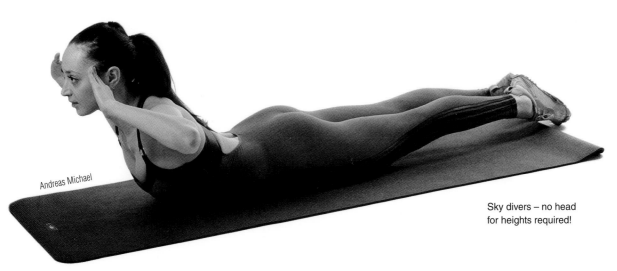

Andreas Michael

Sky divers – no head for heights required!

Total body/cardio

This group of exercises represents the most time-effective movements that you can perform. Do you need to get a lot done in a very brief time? Then these are the exercises for you! Because they utilize multiple muscle groups at the same time, the exercises listed in this final category also have a big impact on your cardiovascular function. Don't be surprised if, after a hard set of burpees or sprinting, your heart rate is higher than it has ever been before...

Note – the following exercises are deemed to be whole-body. While, in most cases, the lower body is providing the majority of the force produced, the arms, core, shoulders, back and chest are also often involved, albeit to a relatively low level in some exercises.

Burpees

Targets: whole body

How to perform: stand with your feet together and your hands by your sides (1). Squat down and place your hands on the floor by your feet (2). Jump your feet back and into the press-up position (3). Perform a single perfect press-up. Jump your feet back up to your hands (4). Leap up into the air as high as you can. Land on slightly bent knees (5) and then immediately drop into another repetition.

Hints, tips and variations: for an easier workout, omit the press-up and/or jump. For variety, add a 180 degree turn to the jump or jump for length rather than height.

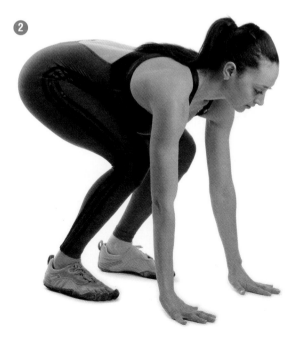

Andreas Michael

No Gym? No problem!

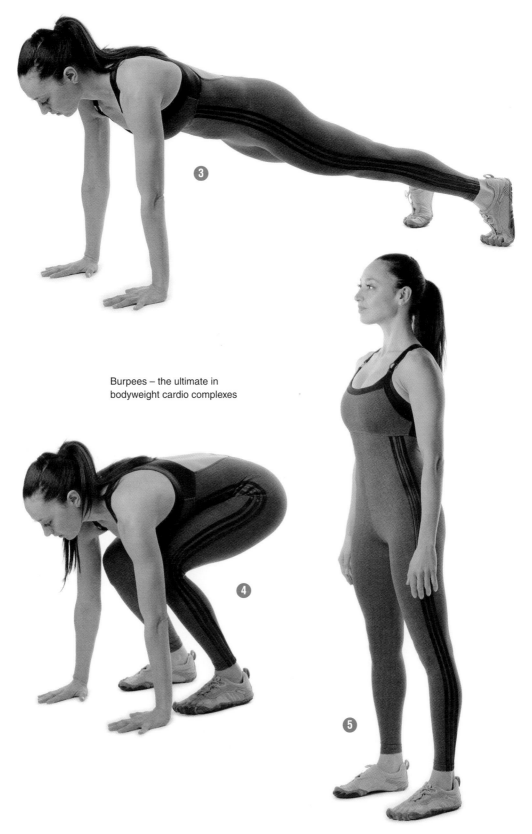

Burpees – the ultimate in
bodyweight cardio complexes

Andreas Michael

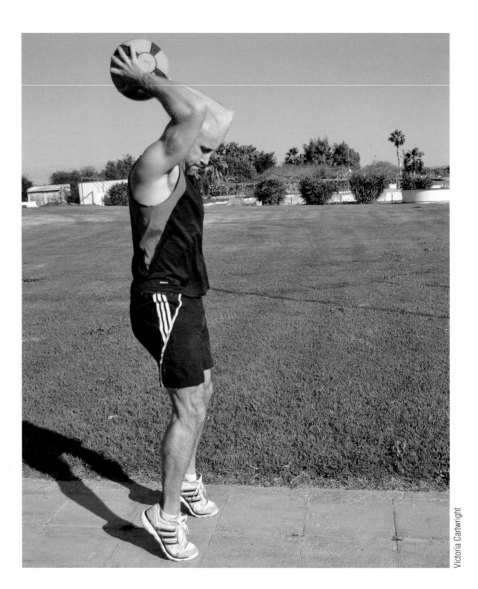

Medicine-ball slams – a great exercise and stress-buster!

Victoria Cartwright

Medicine-ball slams

Targets: whole body

Equipment: medicine ball

How to perform: stand with a medicine ball in your hands and your feet shoulder-width apart. Raise the ball above your head. Using your entire body, hurl the medicine ball down at the floor around 2 ft/60 cm in front of your feet. Catch it as it rebounds and use this momentum as you lift it above your head to repeat.

Hints, tips and variations: add an element of rotation by turning your body and throwing the ball down just to the side of your foot. Alternate sides for the duration of your set.

No Gym? No problem!

Power cleans

Targets: whole body

Equipment: barbell, dumb-bells, kettlebells, sandbag, rock or medicine ball

How to perform: with a weight at your feet, squat down and grasp the weight with an overhand or neutral grip. Lift your chest, tightly arch your lower back and straighten your arms. Explode upwards with your legs and, as the weight approaches waist-height, add a powerful pull with your arms. Drive your elbows forwards so you catch the weight across the front of your shoulders. Roll the weight down the front of your body, lower it to the ground and repeat.

Hints, tips and variations: this exercise can be performed with a barbell, dumb-bells, kettlebells, a sandbag, a big rock or even a medicine ball. Although your hand position may change out of necessity, the lifting action should remain unchanged.

Tyre flips

Targets: whole body

Equipment: tyre

How to perform: squat down next to your tyre with your feet shoulder-width apart. Grasp the underside of the tyre. Using your legs and arms together, stand up and push the tyre so it tips over. Take a step forwards, squat down and repeat.

Hints, tips and variations: instead of merely taking a step after your tyre, perform a two-footed jump into the centre and then out again. Quickly jog back around the tyre and flip again. This exercise can be performed for distance or repetitions.

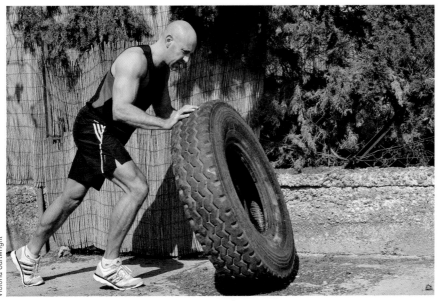

Victoria Cartwright

Andreas Michael

Power cleans – total body strength training

Do not round your back when performing this exercise

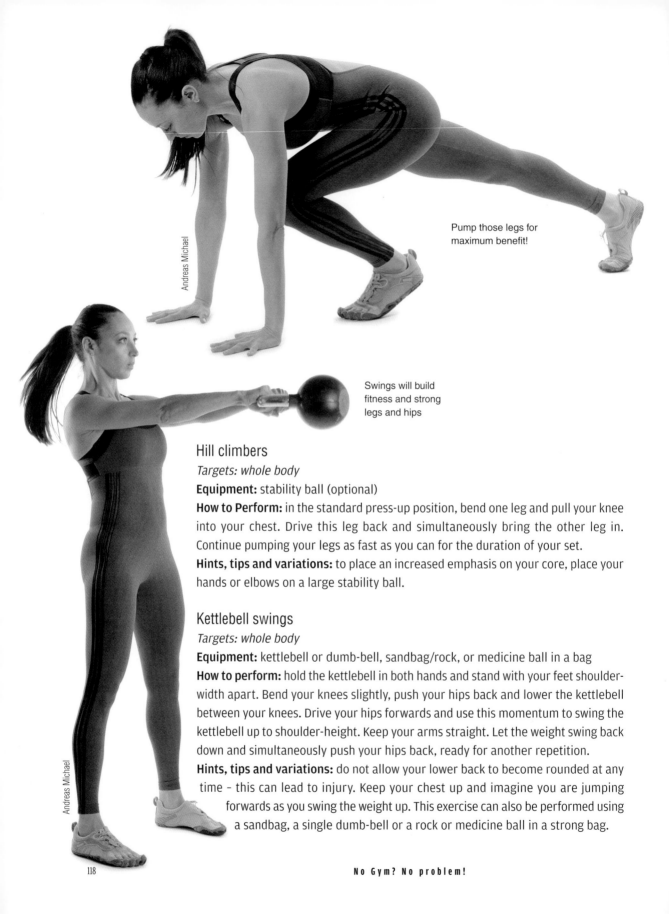

Andreas Michael

Pump those legs for maximum benefit!

Swings will build fitness and strong legs and hips

Hill climbers

Targets: whole body

Equipment: stability ball (optional)

How to Perform: in the standard press-up position, bend one leg and pull your knee into your chest. Drive this leg back and simultaneously bring the other leg in. Continue pumping your legs as fast as you can for the duration of your set.

Hints, tips and variations: to place an increased emphasis on your core, place your hands or elbows on a large stability ball.

Kettlebell swings

Targets: whole body

Equipment: kettlebell or dumb-bell, sandbag/rock, or medicine ball in a bag

How to perform: hold the kettlebell in both hands and stand with your feet shoulder-width apart. Bend your knees slightly, push your hips back and lower the kettlebell between your knees. Drive your hips forwards and use this momentum to swing the kettlebell up to shoulder-height. Keep your arms straight. Let the weight swing back down and simultaneously push your hips back, ready for another repetition.

Hints, tips and variations: do not allow your lower back to become rounded at any time – this can lead to injury. Keep your chest up and imagine you are jumping forwards as you swing the weight up. This exercise can also be performed using a sandbag, a single dumb-bell or a rock or medicine ball in a strong bag.

Andreas Michael

No Gym? No problem!

Thrusters

Targets: whole body

Equipment: barbell, dumb-bells, sandbag, medicine ball, kettlebells or rock

How to perform: stand with your feet shoulder-width apart and hold a weight in front of your shoulders. Push your hips back and bend your knees; squat down until your thighs are roughly parallel to the floor. Stand up with power behind the movement and use this momentum to help you drive the weight up and overhead to arm's length. Lower the weight back to shoulder-height and repeat.

Hints, tips and variations: this exercise can be performed using a barbell, dumb-bells, a sandbag, a medicine ball, kettlebells or a rock.

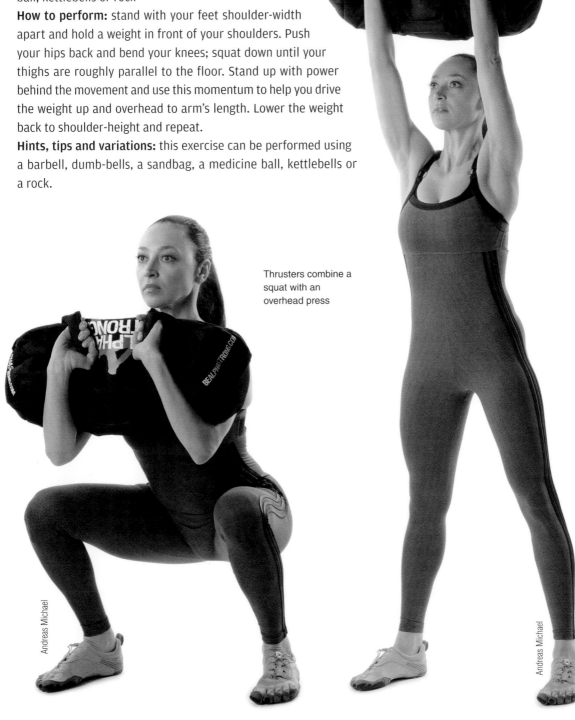

Thrusters combine a squat with an overhead press

Andreas Michael

Andreas Michael

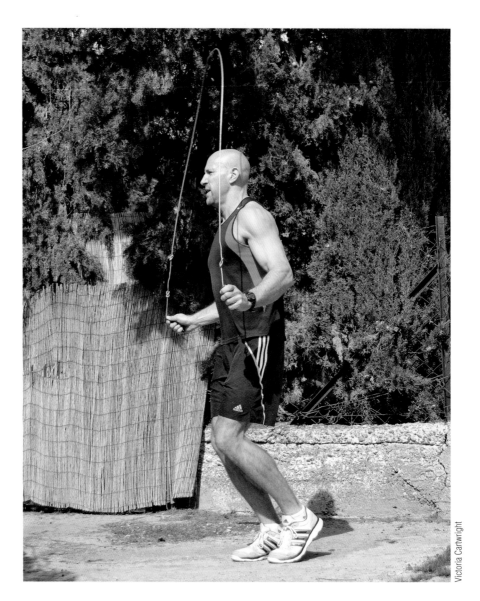

Skipping – not just for schoolgirls!

Victoria Cartwright

Skipping

Targets: whole body

Equipment: skipping rope

How to perform: stand with your feet together on the centre of your skipping rope; the handles should just reach your armpits. Skip using any style you can maintain: feet together, heel/toe 'boxer' skip, running on the spot, high knees or double-unders (two rope turns per jump) (see pages 46-7).

Hints, tips and variations: skipping takes practice but once learnt is an excellent no-frills cardio option. If you are unable to skip, replicate the movement using an imaginary rope.

Sprinting

Targets: whole body

How to perform: when sprinting, make sure you are up on the balls of your feet and leaning slightly forwards. Pump your arms but make sure that your upper body stays relaxed. Avoid clenching your fists or gritting your teeth. Minimize ground contact and aim for fast, light feet.

Hints, tips and variations: sprints can be performed just about anywhere - on a track, the beach, the park, a quiet street, up hills or on the flat. Make sure your

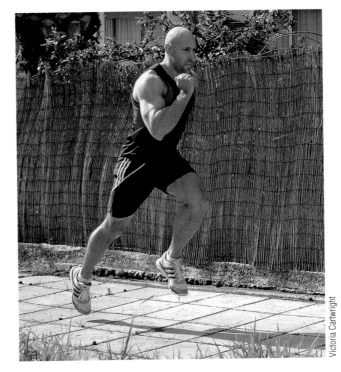

Victoria Cartwright

sprinting surface is smooth to avoid tripping hazards. Warm up thoroughly before sprinting to minimize your risk of injury. Treadmills do not go fast enough for true sprints so do your sprints outdoors for maximum benefit.

Run like you stole it!

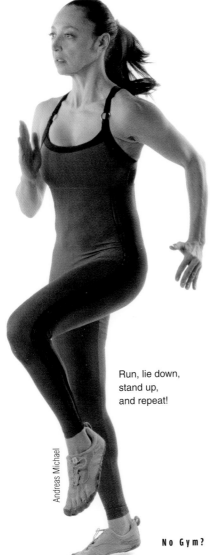

Run, lie down, stand up, and repeat!

Andreas Michael

Sprawls

Targets: whole body

Equipment: exercise mat

How to perform: jog on the spot, keeping your upper body relaxed. Drop to the floor and sprawl onto your stomach with your legs and arms stretched out in an X shape. Get up as fast as you can and continue running.

Hints, tips and variations: sprawls can be performed while running forwards, backwards or sideways as well as on your back.

Bear crawls/crab crawls

Targets: whole body

How to perform: crouch down and place your hands on the floor. Spread your weight evenly fore and aft and 'run' bear-style on all fours for the required distance or time. Keep your abs tight and your head up so you can see where you are going. For crab crawls, simply turn over and perform the same movement but facing skywards instead. Try to push your hips up as you move.

Hints, tips and variations: these exercises can be performed uphill, downhill and even (carefully) up and down stairs.

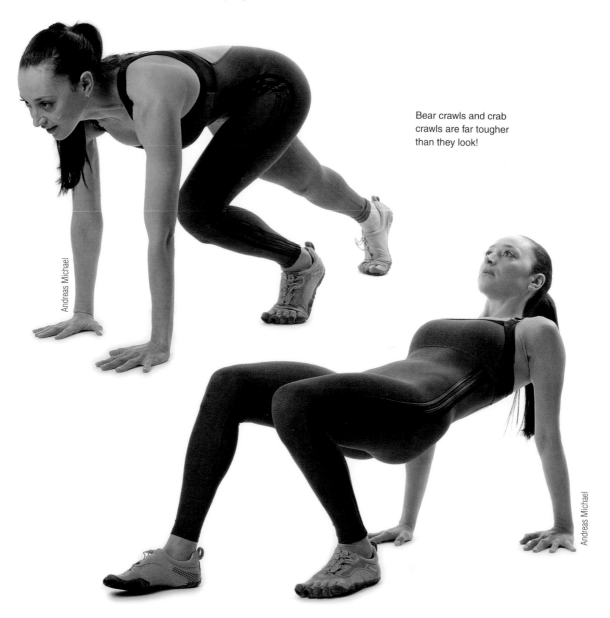

Bear crawls and crab crawls are far tougher than they look!

Andreas Michael

Andreas Michael

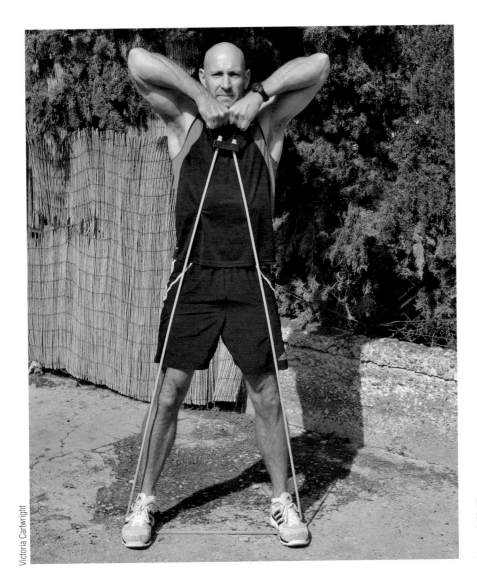

Victoria Cartwright

High-pulls can be
performed with
weights or a
resistance band
as preferred

Band high-pulls

Targets: whole body

Equipment: resistance band, a barbell, dumb-bells, a rock or a sandbag

How to perform: with the middle of your resistance band beneath your feet, stand in a wide stance. With both ends of the band clasped firmly in your hands, bend your knees and squat down. Keep your chest up and your hips low. Stand up with power behind the movement and pull your hands up and under your chin. Your elbows should be higher than your hands. Lower the band and then bend your legs to return to the starting position.

Hints, tips and variations: high-pulls can also be performed with a barbell, an upended dumb-bell, a sandbag, a kettlebell, a big rock or any similarly heavy object.

CHAPTER SIX

Warming up and cooling down

Warming up

As a fledgling Marine, I was often told that Prior Planning and Preparation Prevents Poor Performance. Before every patrol and every operation we planned our tactics and manoeuvres in fine detail to ensure that everything went as smoothly as possible. Failure to plan, they say, means planning to fail and failure is an F word that no Marine wanted to hear!

Just as prior preparation increases the odds of success in military operations, you need to take certain steps to ensure the success of your workouts and that means warming up properly. A warm-up should ensure your mind and body are ready for the workout to come and, as well as increasing your performance potential, a well-designed warm-up should minimize your risk of suffering an injury.

Most of us lead relatively sedentary lives and spend a lot of our work and leisure time sat down. All this sitting means that our muscles tend to shorten and our joints sort of 'dry up' and become less mobile. This is because the lubricating substance that keeps our joints supple, called synovial fluid, is produced on demand and so, if you don't move much, your joints tend to be under-lubricated. Leaping into a high-octane workout with tight muscles and dry joints is a sure fire recipe for injury.

There are numerous warm-up methods and routines that you can choose from but, in my opinion, the two routines I have provided below are the most straightforward and effective. Feel free to use your own warm-up routine – as long as you feel ready to work out you know it's been effective. But, whatever you do, please ensure that you do warm up and don't skip this vital part of your workout. If you think that skipping a few minutes warming up means you are saving time then think again. A warm-up only need take a few minutes and could prevent an injury that halts your workouts for many months or even permanently, so it's time well spent.

Warm-up routine one

Pulse raiser

Perform five to ten minutes of progressively challenging cardio that leaves you warm, gradually elevates your breathing and heart rate and increases blood flow around your body. In addition, this part of your warm-up will also increase synovial fluid production within your joints.

What does progressively challenging mean? Simply start slow and easy and build up gradually until, as you near the end of your pulse raise, your breathing and heart rate are sufficiently elevated that you feel moderately out of breath but still comfortable. Using the perceived exertion scale, you should be hitting around five or six out of ten or an age-adjusted heart rate of around sixty per cent.

Suitable warm-up activities include walking progressing to jogging/running, step-ups and skipping.

Dynamic stretches

Contrary to popular methodology, stretching does not have to be a static activity, especially in a warm-up. You've just spent five to ten minutes getting your heart rate and body temperature up so it makes little sense to spend a further five or so minutes standing still so you get cold and your heart rate drops all the way back down again.

Dynamic stretches are designed to take your muscles and joints through a full range of movement and are basically stretches 'on the go'. There are five exercises in this sequence; perform ten to fifteen repetitions of each one and move from one exercise to the next without pausing to maintain your elevated heart rate and body temperature. On particularly cold days or after lengthy periods of being immobile, it may be a good idea to repeat the sequence two or even three times before moving on to more energetic activities (see photographs on pages 126-8).

1. Squat to overhead reach and twist
2. Push, pull and step back
3. Pull and twist
4. Lunge with a twist
5. Step over and duck under

Squat to overhead reach and twist

With your feet shoulder-width apart and your hands by your sides, squat down and then stand up. As you rise, lift your arms above your head and make yourself as tall as you can. Once you are fully upright, add a small twist to mobilize your spine and waist. Lower your arms, square your shoulders and repeat. Try to increase the depth of your squat as your joints and muscles begin to loosen up.

Warm up your body with squat, reach and twists

A great stretch before running

Push, pull and step back

Stand with your feet together and your arms extended in front of you at shoulder-height. Pull your hands back and into the sides of your chest and simultaneously step back, pushing your heel to the floor to gently stretch your calf. Bring your feet back together and extend your arms again. Repeat but step back with your opposite leg.

Andreas Michael

Andreas Michael

Pull and twist

Stand with your feet together and arms extended in front of you at shoulder-height. Keeping your arms up and perpendicular to the floor, pull your left arm back and simultaneously reach further forwards with your right as you twist your upper body though ninety degrees. Then pull your right arm back, push your left arm forwards and twist in the opposite direction. Imagine you are pulling a rope in towards you. Keep your elbows high and your knees slightly bent throughout.

This exercise warms you up and improves your balance

Imagine you are pulling on a rope...

Andreas Michael

Lunge with a twist

With your feet together and your hands lightly touching your temples, take a large step forwards and bend your legs so your rear knee comes within a couple of inches of the floor. Simultaneously rotate your upper body towards your leading knee. Return to the starting position and repeat on the opposite side.

Andreas Michael

No Gym? No problem!

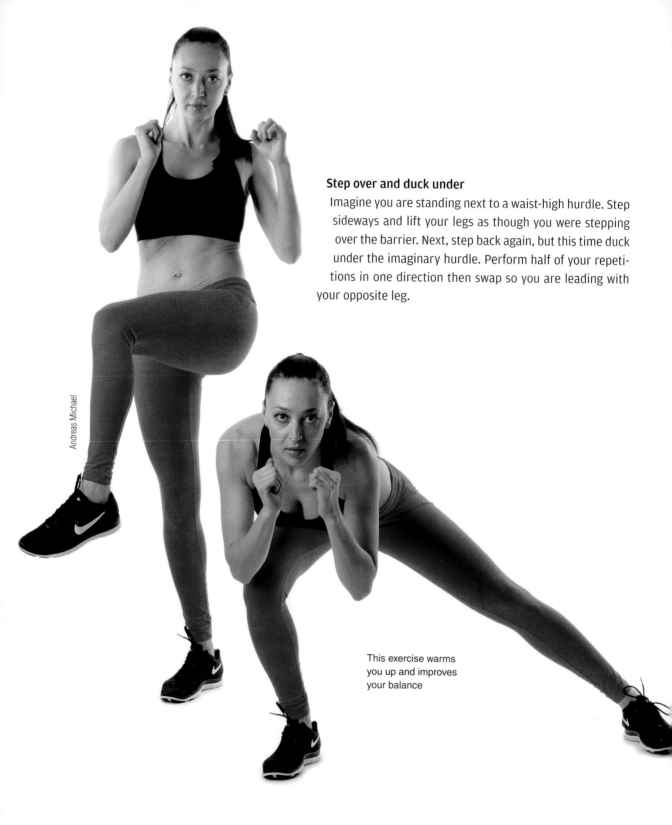

Step over and duck under

Imagine you are standing next to a waist-high hurdle. Step sideways and lift your legs as though you were stepping over the barrier. Next, step back again, but this time duck under the imaginary hurdle. Perform half of your repetitions in one direction then swap so you are leading with your opposite leg.

Andreas Michael

This exercise warms you up and improves your balance

Warm-up routine two

I can't take credit for this routine as it's merely a westernized version of a series of yogic exercises commonly called the sun-salutation sequence. The beauty of this routine is that it involves an element of pulse raising with mobility and dynamic flexibility, all in one. It might take you a while to learn this sequence but, once mastered, it is an all but perfect way to warm up without the use of exercise equipment. Saying that, a mat may make this routine more comfortable, but make sure it is a thin mat that will not move. Sticky yoga mats are obviously ideal.

To make this sequence especially effective, it is important that you only breathe through your nose. This will elevate your heart rate and increase your temperature more noticeably than with mouth breathing. Each exercise in the sequence is performed with a corresponding inhalation or exhalation. If you can, try to make sure you are breathing in or out as detailed but, if you get muddled, don't worry and just continue breathing in time with your movements. Where no breath is indicated, hold your breath until you move into the next position. See photographs on pages 130-31.

1. Stand with your feet together and your hands by your sides. Lift your chest, extend your neck, pull your shoulders back and think tall thoughts!
2. Raise your arms above your head. (INHALE)
3. Bend your knees as far as necessary, hinge forwards through your hips and place your hands on the floor. (EXHALE)
4. Bend your knees and drop down into a crouch.
5. Jump your feet back lightly and into the classic press-up position.
6. Lower your chest down towards the floor. (INHALE)
7. Keeping your hips down, extend your arms and lift your chest up as far as your back flexibility allows. (EXHALE) Lower your chest back to the floor. (INHALE)
8. Keeping your body straight and tight, extend your arms and come back up into a triangular position. (EXHALE)
9. Step your right leg up to your hands and into a lunge position. (INHALE)
10. Step in with your left leg into a crouch position. (EXHALE)
11. Stand up and simultaneously raise your arms above your head. (INHALE)
12. Lower your arms to your sides. (EXHALE)
13. Repeat entire series of steps but use the opposite leg in movements 9 and 10.

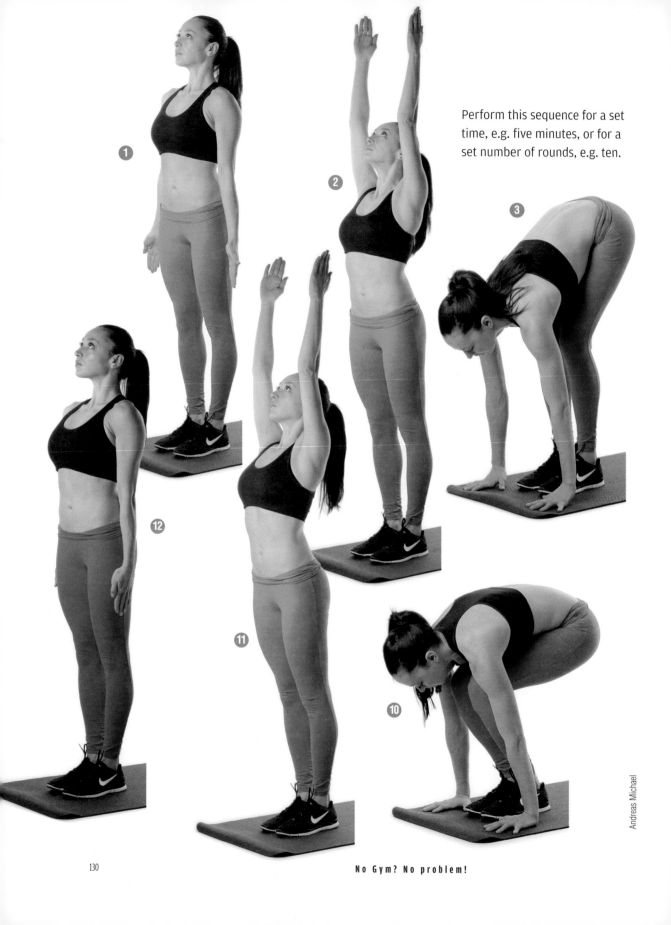

Perform this sequence for a set time, e.g. five minutes, or for a set number of rounds, e.g. ten.

No Gym? No problem!

Andreas Michael

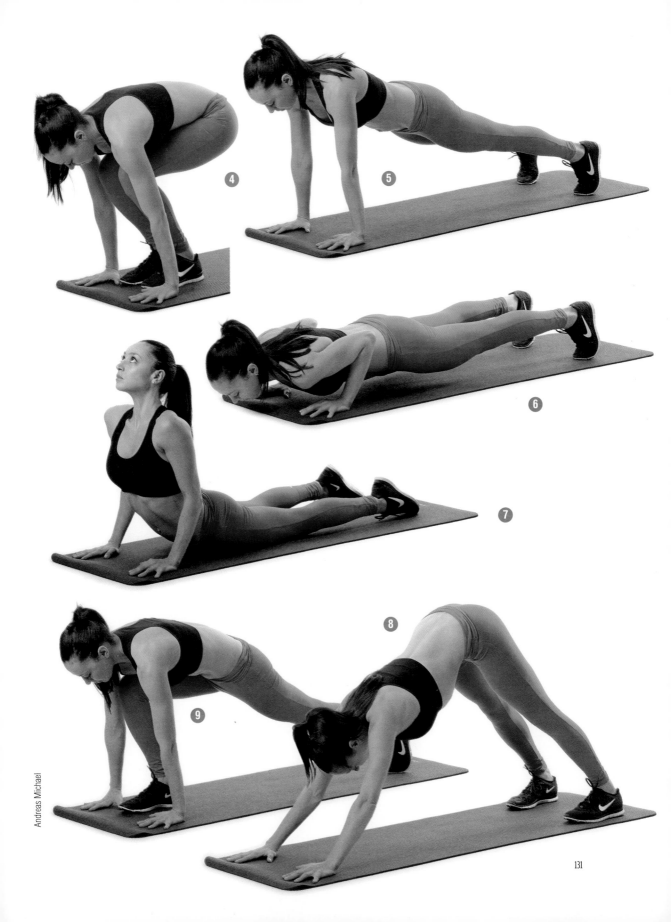

131

Cooling down

Once your workout is complete, it's time to cool down. The cool-down can really test your workout discipline as it's very tempting to just collapse in a heap after training or head straight for the shower, glad that you have finished your workout for the day. Cool-downs are designed to return your body to its pre-exercise state – a condition called homeostasis, which literally means hormonally balanced. You must return your body to homeostasis for the recovery process to begin.

In addition to kick-starting the recovery process, cool-downs promote flexibility and can also reduce the severity and duration of post-exercise muscle soreness. A cool-down consists of two phases: a pulse lowerer and stretches.

Pulse lowerer

The purpose of the pulse lowerer is to promote venous return and help supply your hard-worked muscles with freshly re-oxygenated blood. When you exercise, blood pools within your working muscles and, with it, the waste products of metabolism accumulate. Flushing your muscles through with freshly oxygenated blood helps clear these metabolic remnants away and promotes recovery. A pulse lowerer is merely the reversal of the pulse raiser performed in your warm-up; perform some cardio at a reasonable level of intensity and then reduce your speed over three to five minutes. You should finish your pulse lowerer when your breathing is approaching normal and you feel ready to do some stretching.

Stretches

The dynamic stretches performed in the warm-up are great at preparing your muscles for exercise but not so good for improving or maintaining your flexibility. Flexibility, also known as suppleness, is the range of movement available at your joints and is an important, if often overlooked, fitness component.

A better choice for your cool-down is static stretches. Static stretches, as the name implies, are stretches that are held for time rather than performed for repetitions. There are two main types of static stretch: maintenance and developmental.

Maintenance stretches are held for ten to twenty seconds and are designed to stop you losing your flexibility. This type of stretching is ideal if you already have good flexibility. Developmental stretches are held for thirty to sixty seconds or more and are used when you want to improve your flexibility. Your cool-down may contain one or both types of stretching depending on your current flexibility requirements.

To save you having to design your own cool-down, just perform the following stretches after each and every workout. Hold the stretches for as long as you deem necessary based on your flexibility. As a general rule, if the muscle you are stretching feels tight, hold the stretch for longer.

Standing calf stretch

Stand at arm's length from a wall or post and place your hands out at shoulder-level. Step your left leg back and bend your right knee. Press your left heel into the floor ensuring that your ankle, knee and hip are aligned and your left foot is pointing straight at the wall. Keep your head and chest up for the duration of the stretch. Change legs and repeat.

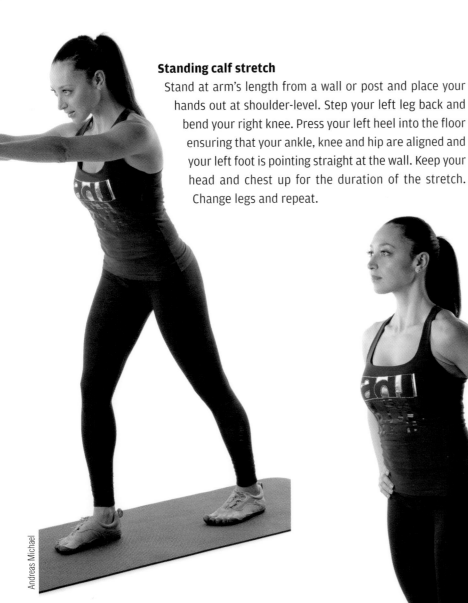

Andreas Michael

Standing quad stretch

Perform this stretch next to a wall or post if you need help with balance. Bend your left leg behind you and grasp around your ankle with your left hand. Point your left knee down at the floor and keep your legs together. Pull your left foot towards your bottom. Hold this position while maintaining an upright torso. On completion, change legs and repeat.

Andreas Michael

Standing hamstring stretch

Place your left leg on a knee-high box, bench or step. Lean forwards from the hips and gently lower your chest towards your left thigh. Bend your right leg slightly to aid in balance and place your hands on your left thigh. Increase the stretch by pushing your bottom back, not by rounding your upper back. Change legs and repeat.

Kneeling forearm stretch

Kneel down and place your fingertips on the floor with your palms facing away from you. Gently press your palms down onto the floor and gently rock back onto your heels. This is an intense stretch so ease into it gradually. Tight forearms are not uncommon so don't be surprised if you have limited movement in this exercise.

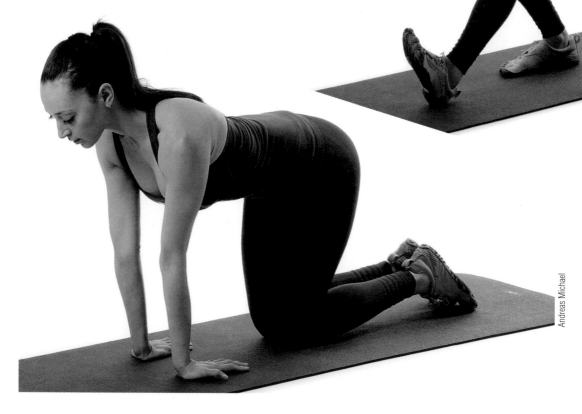

Andreas Michael

Andreas Michael

Kneeling hip flexor stretch

Kneel down on the floor and then take a large step forwards so that your front shin is vertical and your rear leg is extended behind you, with your knee placed on the floor. Keep your body upright. Relax and sink your hips down towards the floor. Slide your rear leg further back as necessary. Place your hands on your front thigh and hold this position for the required duration. Come out of the stretch slowly, change legs and repeat.

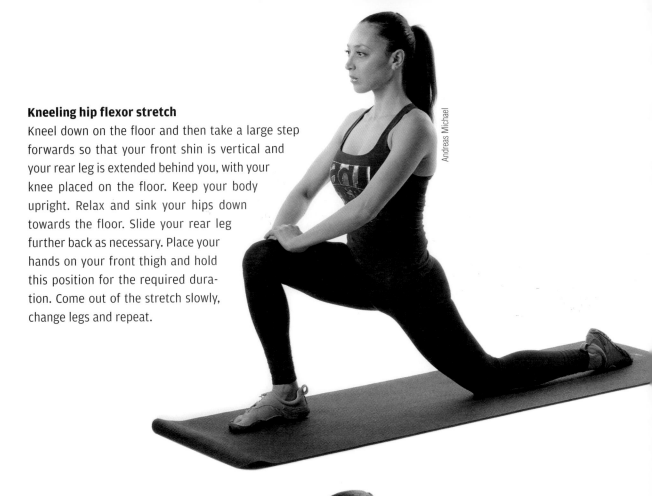

Andreas Michael

Seated groin stretch

Sit on the floor with the soles of your feet together and your legs bent. Draw your feet as close as possible to your groin. Wrap your hands around your ankles and place your elbows on your legs. Use your arms to gently push your knees down towards the floor if required.

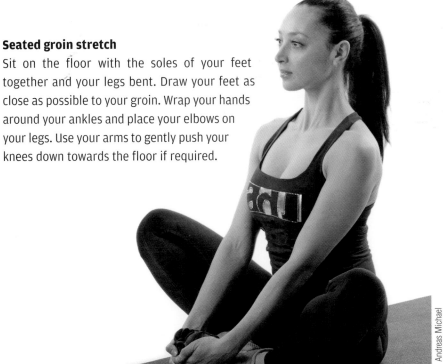

Andreas Michael

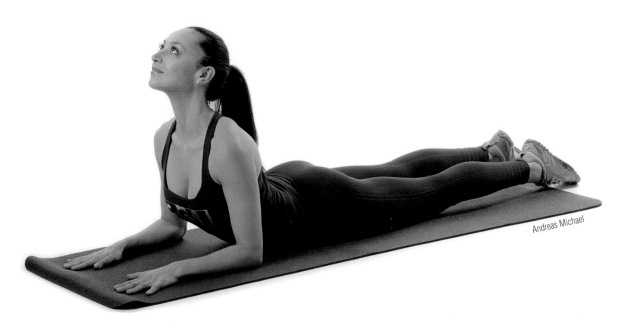

Andreas Michael

Lying ab stretch

Lie on your front with your arms bent, your forearms flat on the floor and your hands extended in front of you. Imagine you are reading a book while lying on a beach! Lift your chest and hold this position for the required length of time. Keep your hips on the floor and your legs straight throughout this stretch.

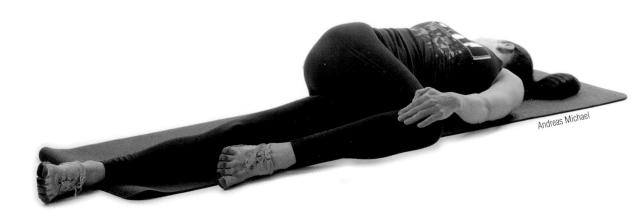

Andreas Michael

Lying glute stretch with spinal twist

Lie on your back with your legs straight and your hands by your sides. Bend your right leg and place your foot next to your left knee. Put your right arm on the floor at shoulder-height and reach your left arm across your body, grasping the outside of your right knee. Roll your lower body to the left, keeping your right arm flat on the floor. Hold this position for the desired duration before slowly returning to the centre and repeating the stretch on the other side.

No Gym? No problem!

Standing chest stretch

Stand up straight and place your hands on your lower back. Keeping your torso upright, push your elbows back to stretch your chest and shoulders. For a more challenging stretch, you can extend your arms as shown in the second image.

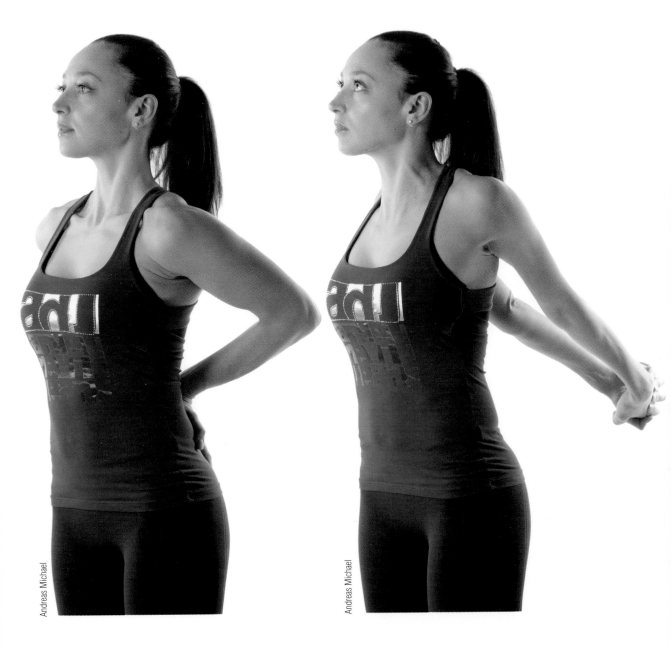

Andreas Michael

Andreas Michael

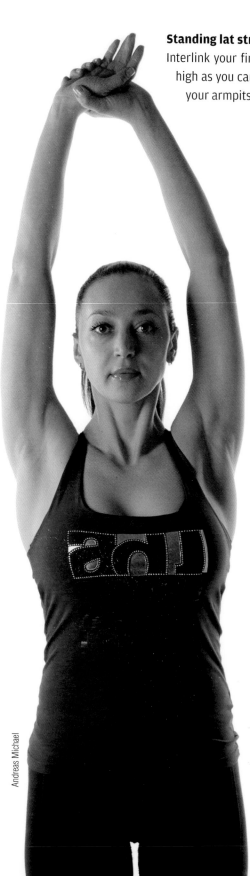

Andreas Michael

Standing lat stretch

Interlink your fingers and press your arms up and overhead. Reach up as high as you can. You should feel a mild stretch in your sides and beneath your armpits. Lean slightly to each side to increase the depth of stretch.

Seven tips for better stretching

1. Only stretch your muscles when they are warm - stretching cold muscles may lead to injury.
2. Do not bounce! Bouncing when stretching is dangerous and can result in injury.
3. Stay relaxed when stretching - do not let your shoulders, jaw, neck or hands tense up as this will reduce the effectiveness of your stretch.
4. Breathe! Exhale as you relax into a stretch. Holding your breath will only impair your stretch.
5. If you are really inflexible, consider stretching every day - possibly twice or more for particularly stiff muscles. If it has taken you years to stiffen up it'll take more than a few minutes a week to make you flexible again!
6. If you find it difficult to find the time to stretch after your workout - maybe because you are hungry or in a rush to get to work - just perform a few maintenance stretches after exercising and then have a proper stretch when it's more conven-ient, e.g. when watching the TV at the end of your day.
7. Never force a stretch; if you feel any burning or your muscles are shaking uncontrollably you are overdoing it so back off before you hurt yourself.

CHAPTER SEVEN

Programme templates

I n Chapter 8 I will provide you with fifteen of my favourite no-frills general-training workouts. However, if you have more specific fitness goals, you may need to design your own bespoke training sessions and, in this chapter, I've provided you with a number of ready-to-use workout templates into which you can plug your favourite exercises. In four weeks or so, simply change the template you are following or, alternatively, stick with the same template but select different exercises.

Adjust the workouts to meet your fitness goals. If you want to develop muscular endurance, select exercises that allow you to perform a high number of repetitions before you become fatigued. Alternatively, if you want to increase your strength, the exercises should be difficult enough to prevent you from performing high repetitions.

Training goal	Repetition range	Recovery between sets
Endurance	12–20+	30–60 seconds
Hypertrophy (muscle size)	6–12	60–90 seconds
Strength	1–5	120–180 seconds

All the exercises used as examples in the following workouts are described in detail in the exercise library in Chapter 5.

Whole-body workout

Perform two to three times a week on non-consecutive days

	Exercise classification	Example exercise
1	Leg exercise	Squats
2	Upper-body push	Press-ups
3	Upper-body pull	Pull-ups
4	Leg exercise	Wrestler squats
5	Upper-body push	1½ side lateral raises
6	Upper-body pull	Isometric towel row
7	Core exercise	Sky divers
8	Core exercise	Side planks

Two-way split routine

Perform once a week, e.g. Monday

	Exercise classification	Example exercise
1	Leg exercise	Squat jumps
2	Leg exercise	One-legged Romanian deadlifts
3	Leg exercise	Supine hip bridges
4	Core exercise	Reverse crunches
5	Core exercise	Sky divers

Perform once a week, e.g. Thursday

	Exercise classification	Example exercise
1	Upper-body push	Handstand press-ups
2	Upper-body pull	Chin-ups
3	Upper-body push	Band side lateral raises
4	Upper-body pull	Isometric towel shrugs
5	Upper-body push	Pike press-ups
6	Upper-body pull	Eccentric pull-ups

Four-way split routine

Perform once a week, e.g. Monday

	Exercise classification	Example exercise
1	Upper-body push	Plyometric press-ups
2	Upper-body pull	Towel pull-ups
3	Upper-body push	Staggered hand press-ups
4	Upper-body pull	Isometric towel shrugs
5	Upper-body push	1½ side lateral raises
6	Upper-body pull	Eccentric pull-ups

Perform once a week, e.g. Tuesday

	Exercise classification	Example exercise
1	Leg exercise	Rear foot elevated split squats
2	Leg exercise	Lunges
3	Leg exercise	Squat crunches
4	Core exercise	Reverse crunches
5	Core exercise	Stability-ball back extentions

Perform once a week, e.g. Thursday

	Exercise classification	Example exercise
1	Upper-body push	Diamond press-ups
2	Upper-body pull	Climber pull-ups
3	Upper-body push	Isometric chest press
4	Upper-body pull	Body rows
5	Upper-body push	Dips
6	Upper-body pull	Towel pull-downs

No Gym? No problem!

Perform once a week, e.g. Friday

	Exercise classification	Example exercise
1	Leg exercise	Jumping lunges
2	Leg exercise	Step-ups
3	Leg exercise	Isometric chest press
4	Core exercise	Reverse crunches
5	Core exercise	Seated Russian twists

Peripheral Heart Action fat-loss workout circuit

Perform two to three times a week on non-consecutive days

	Exercise classification	Example exercise
1	Leg exercise	Squats
2	Upper-body push	Pike press-ups
3	Leg exercise	Lunges
4	Upper-body pull	Towel pull-downs
5	Whole-body exercise	Burpees
6	Leg exercise	Jumping lunges
7	Upper-body push	Dips
8	Leg exercise	One-legged Romanian deadlifts
9	Upper-body pull	Body rows
10	Whole-body exercise	Sprawls

CHAPTER EIGHT

Sample workouts

Sometimes it's nice to disengage your brain and follow a pre-designed workout. While this does mean that you will be following a workout that wasn't specifically designed for you, it also means you can simply turn up and work out without having to do too much planning or preparation.

With any pre-prescribed workout, feel free to make modifications based on your personal level of fitness, injury history and exercise experience. Don't be a slave to any prescribed workout and risk injury when a few simple changes can make your entire workout experience more enjoyable and rewarding.

Note – always warm up before and cool down after each workout and remember that rest days and good nutrition are equally as important as training hard! All the exercises detailed in the programme below are explained in the exercise library in Chapter 5.

The running burpee pyramid workout

This workout is as basic as it gets. All you need is about 20 m of space and, if you want a more comfortable option, an exercise mat, although a pair of gloves to keep your hands warm and dry will suffice. This workout will test local muscular endurance and also your cardiovascular fitness. Take it easy on the runs until you get a feel for the intensity of the workout.

Place two markers around 20 m apart. Don't worry too much about the exact distance. Measure out twenty-five strides and you'll be close enough for our purposes.

Follow this sequence from top to bottom, only resting once you have completed the walking lunges...

- Run out, perform 5 burpees and then run back.
- Run out, perform 5 burpees and 10 press-ups and then run back.
- Run out, perform 5 burpees, 10 press-ups, 15 squats and then run back.
- Run out, perform 5 burpees, 10 press-ups, 15 squats, 20 hill climbers and then run back.
- Run out, perform 5 burpees, 10 press-ups, 15 squats, 20 hill climbers and then perform walking lunges back to the start.
- Rest and then repeat from the beginning.

Beginners – 2–3 laps, rest 2 minutes between laps
Intermediate – 4–6 laps, rest 90 seconds between laps
Advanced – 7–10 laps, rest 60 seconds between laps

You can also adjust the repetitions to suit your individual fitness level, for example, by performing three, six, nine and twelve repetitions of the exercises respectively. Also, feel free to walk or jog between markers or shorten the distance.

50/40/30/20/10 descending rep circuit

This workout is designed to be all-encompassing, combining muscular endurance exercises for every major muscle group with a significant cardiovascular challenge. It's against the clock so you can pace yourself according to your current personal fitness level. Feel free to adjust the suggested repetition ranges up or down as necessary and by all means make exercise substitutions but try to remain true to the spirit of the workout by selecting similar exercises.

Start your watch and perform fifty repetitions of each exercise in the following sequence. On reaching the last exercise, repeat the sequence, but only perform forty repetitions. Continue working your way through the sequence, but drop ten reps from the count each time until your final round consists of ten reps per exercise. Rest when you need to but try and keep going as the clock is ticking right up to the very end!

1. Press-ups
2. Squats
3. Crunches
4. Body rows
5. Jumping jacks

Three-minute rounds

For this workout, simply perform as many repetitions of each of the following exercises as possible in thirty seconds. Move from one exercise to the next without pausing and only rest when you have completed the sixth exercise. This totals three minutes. Rest for one minute and then repeat. I like to do five rounds of this workout to total twenty minutes, but please feel free to adjust the number of rounds performed according to your personal fitness level.

As you get fitter, you can make this workout more demanding by taking a few seconds off your recovery, adding a few seconds to the rounds or simply increasing the number of rounds performed.

Use a programmable timer or, keep an eye on the sweep hand of a clock. Feel free to select different exercises but try to stay true to the spirit of the workout, i.e. swap a leg exercise for a leg exercise. Remember, you are only performing thirty seconds of each exercise so don't hang about on your transitions and try to really crank out the reps. The muscles you have just used will get a rest during the following specifically sequenced exercise.

1. Skipping
2. Press-ups
3. Squats
4. Chinnies
5. Towel pull-downs
6. Burpees

Tabata interval circuit

For this workout you'll need a programmable timer such as a Gymboss: alternatively, there are lots of smartphone apps available that work just as well. If you don't have access to either of these options, you can perform this workout by keeping an eye on the sweep hand of a well-placed clock. You'll also need a skipping rope, an exercise mat and a little bit of space.

Perform twenty seconds of each exercise in sequence and use the ten-second recovery to move to the next exercise. There are four exercises in the circuit and you should perform eight to ten laps in total - so sixteen to twenty minutes for the entire workout. Place the exercises close together so you don't waste any time in the transitions.

1. Skipping - knee-lift sprints
2. Press-ups
3. Chinnies
4. Squats

So your workout will look like this:

- 20 seconds skipping
- 10 seconds rest/transition
- 20 seconds press-ups
- 10 seconds rest/transition
- 20 seconds chinnies
- 10 seconds rest/transition
- 20 seconds squats
- 10 seconds rest/transition

Start from the top again with 20 seconds skipping. Repeat for 8 or 10 laps

Workout strategy

True Tabata intervals, as described in Chapter 4 (see pages 81–2), do not allow for pacing – you go as fast as you can for each and every work period. Despite the fact that, by using a variety of muscle groups you are moving the stress around your body, it is unrealistic to perform each of the thirty-plus intervals at maximal effort. I suggest you work hard but just shy of 'eyeballs out' intensity. While this pacing contradicts true Tabata intervals, it will make this workout a challenging undertaking as opposed to an impossible one!

Make a mental note of how many repetitions you manage in your first lap and endeavour to hit similar numbers in each subsequent lap. The next time you perform this workout, try to add a rep or two.

The 'eat the biggest frog first' workout

What is the best way to eat a plate of frogs? Scoff the biggest one first and then it's all downhill from there! This workout follows the same principle. To complete it, you'll need something to do pull-ups from, a stopwatch, a pen and a sheet of paper. Write the repetition counts on page 148 down so you can keep track of your progress. Warm up appropriately with some light cardio, dynamic stretches and joint mobility exercises. In addition, spend a couple of minutes practicing pull-ups, press-ups and squats to ensure your exercise technique is spot on.

The aim of this workout is to storm through all ten sets as fast as you can and complete the workout in the shortest time possible. If you are very fit, this may mean that you take minimal rest between exercises. If you are less fit, you might want to start with a lower number of initial reps or allow yourself to take breaks between sets and even between repetitions. As you get fitter, strive to rest less and work more so, ultimately, this workout becomes a non-stop circuit.

Once you are ready, start your stopwatch and perform ten pull-ups, immediately followed by twenty press-ups and then finally thirty squats. On completion of this triplet, go straight back to the pull-up bar and repeat the sequence but reducing the repetitions as shown. Continue knocking off reps set by set until you finally perform one pull-up, two press-ups and three squats. Stop your watch, note the time and record it for future workouts.

- 10 pull-ups
- 20 press-ups
- 30 squats

- 9 pull-ups
- 18 press-ups
- 27 squats

- 8 pull-ups
- 16 press-ups
- 24 squats

- 7 pull-ups
- 14 press-ups
- 21 pquats

- 6 pull-ups
- 12 press-ups
- 18 squats

- 5 pull-ups
- 10 press-ups
- 15 squats

- 4 pull-ups
- 8 press-ups
- 12 squats

- 3 pull-ups
- 6 press-ups
- 9 squats

- 2 pull-ups
- 4 press-ups
- 6 squats

- 1 pull-up
- 2 press-ups
- 3 squats

No Gym? No problem!

The odds and evens push and pull workout

For this workout you need a bar from which you can perform pull-ups, an exercise mat and a stopwatch.

Warm up thoroughly, paying special attention to your upper body. Make sure your wrists, elbows and shoulders are warm and thoroughly mobilized.

Start your stopwatch and perform as many press-ups as possible – really do your best to pump out the maximum number of repetitions. On completion, make a note of the number of repetitions performed.

Next, at the top of the second minute, perform a maximum number of chin-ups or pull-ups. You can use a palms-under or palms-over grip – it's entirely up to you. As before, perform as many repetitions as possible and then record your score.

At the top of the third minute, perform another maximum-rep set of press-ups. Unless you are some kind of press-up master, you'll perform considerably fewer reps this time around. Make a note of the number of reps performed.

At the top of the following minute, perform another set of pull-ups. Do as many as you can until you are unable to do any more.

Continue alternating between maximum-rep sets of press-ups and pull-ups until you have completed ten sets of each totalling twenty minutes. Add up the total number of press-ups and pull-ups completed and record this total – it's the target to beat the next time you attempt this workout.

To recap – your workout should look like this (AMRAP is short for As Many Reps As Possible):

- 1st minute – AMRAP press-ups
- 2nd minute – AMRAP pull-ups
- 3rd minute – AMRAP press-ups
- 4th minute – AMRAP pull-ups
- 5th minute – AMRAP press-ups
- 6th minute – AMRAP pull-ups
- 7th minute – AMRAP press-ups
- 8th minute – AMRAP pull-ups
- 9th minute – AMRAP press-ups
- 10th minute – AMRAP pull-ups
- 11th minute – AMRAP press-ups
- 12th minute – AMRAP pull-ups
- 13th minute – AMRAP press-ups
- 14th minute – AMRAP pull-ups
- 15th minute – AMRAP press-ups
- 16th minute – AMRAP pull-ups
- 17th minute – AMRAP press-ups
- 18th minute – AMRAP pull-ups

- 19th minute – AMRAP press-ups
- 20th minute – AMRAP pull-ups

Total press-up/pull-up reps = your total score. Try to beat this next time you repeat this workout.

Workout variation

This workout can easily be adapted to become a full-body challenge by simply adding a set of speed squats in between each upper-body exercise...

- 1st minute – AMRAP press-ups
- 3rd minute – AMRAP speed squats
- 2nd minute – AMRAP pull-ups
- 4th minute etc. repeat sequence

This will really crank up your heart rate. If you choose this option, perform seven sets to total twenty-one minutes of work.

The up and down again pyramid workout

All you need for this workout is some space for running, a mat, a pull-up bar, a skipping rope and a stopwatch. Measure out 50 m and place a marker at both ends for easy reference.

Begin the workout by spending three to five minutes warming up. Perform some light cardio, dynamic stretches and joint-mobility exercises and then a few reps of each exercise by way of practice and preparation.

- Run 500 m (10 shuttle runs of 50 m each)
- 10 chin-ups*
- 20 burpees**
- 30 W sits
- 40 skipping double-unders (or 100 regular rope turns)
- 50 squats
- 40 skipping double-unders (or 100 regular rope turns)
- 30 W sits
- 20 burpees**
- 10 chin-ups*
- Run 500 m (10 shuttle runs of 50 m each)

*If you are unable to perform chin-ups, feel free to substitute with body rows.
**If a full burpee (including press-up and jump) is too much for you, simply leave out one or both of these elements.

Ten-minute bodyweight challenge

Short on time but still want a great workout? This one takes exactly ten minutes and is completely equipment-free so it's ideal for hotel rooms or a quick training session at home. Change the exercises to reflect your personal preferences and abilities.

Perform one minute of each of the following:

* Press-ups
* Squats
* Skipping or jumping jacks
* W sits

Follow immediately with forty-five seconds of each of these:

* Press-ups
* Squats
* Skipping or jumping jacks
* W sits

Then thirty seconds of each of the following:

* Press-ups
* Squats
* Skipping or jumping jacks
* W sits

And finally, perform fifteen seconds of each of these:

* Press-ups
* Squats
* Skipping or jumping jacks
* W sits

If you get it right, you should complete ten minutes of non-stop exercise.

Press-up/burpee pyramid

This is another short, sharp workout that gets a lot done in a very short time. Burpees are probably the ultimate total-body exercise as they work your arms, legs and core, as well as providing a great cardio workout. This one starts off easy enough but gets much tougher towards the end...

Perform burpees as per the instructions below but increase the number of press-ups you perform mid-burpee each time.*

- Stand with your feet together and your hands by your sides.
- Bend down and place your hands outside your feet.
- Jump your feet back into the press-up position.
- Perform a single press-up.*
- Jump your feet back in.
- Stand up.

Option 1 - stop at ten press-ups ... your workout is complete!
Option 2 - carry on adding a press-up per burpee until you are unable to continue and see just how many you can do...
Option 3 - on reaching ten press-ups, continue but reduce the press-ups/push-ups by one rep at a time until you get back down to one.

Spartan circuit

This workout has very little to do with Ancient Greek warriors and more to do with a sparseness of equipment. Don't let the simplicity of this workout fool you – it's a very challenging and effective training session.

Perform the exercises listed below as a non-stop circuit. This workout starts with five minutes of skipping so there is no need to spend extra time warming up. All exercises are detailed in the exercise library in Chapter 5.

Set your timer for two minutes of work (in the form of bodyweight exercises) and one minute of recovery (in the form of skipping).

- 2 minutes - skipping (slow to warm up)
- 1 minute - skipping (a little faster)
- 2 minutes - skipping (fast - try to maintain this speed for the rest of the workout)
- 1 minute - squats
- 2 minutes - skipping
- 1 minute - front plank
- 2 minutes - skipping
- 1 minute - press-ups
- 2 minutes - skipping

- 1 minute – lunges
- 2 minutes – skipping
- 1 minute – pike press-ups
- 2 minutes – skipping
- 1 minute – left side plank
- 2 minutes – skipping
- 1 minute – wrestler squats
- 2 minutes – skipping
- 1 minute – diamond press-ups
- 2 minutes – skipping
- 1 minute – right side plank

Deck of cards workouts

Deck of cards workouts are a lot like having your very own personal trainer in your pocket. Simply allocate an exercise to each colour or suit and then follow the instructions below...

Workout one

Red cards = squats

Black cards = press-ups

Jokers = 300 rope turns with the skipping rope

Face value 1-10 = 1-10 reps, so 6 of hearts = 6 squats

Picture cards = 12 reps, so king of spades = 12 press-ups

Workout two

Diamonds = lunges

Hearts = squats

Clubs = hill climbers

Spades = press-ups

Jokers = 1-minute plank

Face value 1-10 = 1-10 reps, so 6 of clubs = 6 hill climbers on each leg

Picture cards = 12 reps, so king of diamonds = 12 lunges on each leg

Shuffle the cards, including the jokers, and place them face down. Work your way through the deck one card at a time. The aim of the game is to get through the pack as fast as possible. If you need to break your sets up with small rests then go ahead, but remember the clock is ticking. Finish all the reps for one card before turning over the next. If you happen to get a run of high cards ... bad luck! Remember that each time a high card comes along, that's one less high rep set you have to do.

Prisoner burpee ladder

This workout is so-called because it can be performed in a space as small as a prison cell! It's a race against the clock so, while it's okay to rest, remember, the clock is ticking...

Work your way down the following descending repetition ladder as fast as you can. Take a breather between each 'rung' but try not to break up the sets of burpees unless absolutely essential – especially towards the end as the reps get lower. Burpee performance is detailed in Chapter 5.

If a twenty-to-one ladder seems a bit daunting, feel free to perform a fifteen-to-one or even a ten-to-one ladder...

- 20 burpees
- 19 burpees
- 18 burpees
- 17 burpees
- 16 burpees
- 15 burpees
- 14 burpees
- 13 burpees
- 12 burpees
- 11 burpees
- 10 burpees
- 9 burpees
- 8 burpees
- 7 burpees
- 6 burpees
- 5 burpees
- 4 burpees
- 3 burpees
- 2 burpees
- 1 burpees

Total – 210 burpees

Legs, legs, legs!

Simple but effective, this lower-body workout should leave your legs weak and your heart pumping!

Perform each group of three exercises as fast as you can and then take the prescribed rest. The first couple of sets should be relatively easy but then, as fatigue sets in and the reps increase, it turns into quite a demanding workout!

- 5 squat jumps
- 5 squats
- 10-second wall squat
- Rest for 30-60 seconds

- 10 squat jumps
- 10 squats
- 20-second wall squat
- Rest for 30-60 seconds

- 15 squat jumps
- 15 squats
- 30-second wall squat
- Rest for 30-60 seconds

- 20 squat jumps
- 20 squats
- 40-second wall squat
- Rest for 30-60 seconds

- 15 squat jumps
- 15 squats
- 30-second wall squat
- Rest for 30-60 seconds

- 10 squat jumps
- 10 squats
- 20-second wall squat
- Rest for 30-60 seconds

- 5 squat jumps
- 5 squats
- 10-second wall squat

Broken 100 m sprints

Sprinting is a great cardio, leg, lung and fat-burning workout, but not everyone has access to a running track or wide open spaces. For this workout, all you need is around 25 m of space.

Find some flat ground, e.g. a quiet car park, a playing field or similar. Place markers 5 m, 10 m, 15 m and 20 m away from your starting point – see diagram below.

5 m ——————————→ 10 m ——————————→ 15 m ——————————→ 20 m

Run out to the first marker as fast as you can and then back to the start, before running straight out to the second marker and back, then to the third marker and back and finally to the fourth marker and back. This totals 100 m. Rest for one to two minutes before repeating for five to eight sets.

For a real challenge, try to perform one broken hundred metres every minute for ten minutes or every ninety seconds for fifteen minutes … the faster you run the more rest you get. You could also do this workout uphill for a totally terrific challenge!

Super-six circuit

This workout will develop muscular endurance and cardiovascular fitness while also burning a whole lot of calories. Much of this calorie burning comes courtesy of EPOC (short for Excessive Post-exercise Oxygen Consumption, which is discussed in Chapter 4, see pages 80–81). In simple terms, EPOC describes how your metabolic rate remains elevated after intense, lactic acid-forming exercise, resulting in greater energy expenditure, even during rest. Think of EPOC as two workouts for the price of one – a real bargain!

Perform the prescribed number of repetitions of each exercise, taking absolutely minimal rest between them; only rest once you have completed the final exercise. Perform as many laps of the circuit as you can in twenty minutes and try to beat your score each time you repeat this workout. For a more challenging workout, simply increase the time and perform more laps.

	Exercise	Repetitions
1	Burpees	12
2	Chinnies	12 per side
3	Box jumps	24
4	Press-ups	12
5	Planks	30 seconds
6	Jumping lunges	12 per leg

CHAPTER NINE

Twelve-week sample exercise plan

There is nothing to stop you putting your own weekly exercise plan together where you alternate strength and cardio training day by day. Such an approach will ensure you develop a respectable level of strength and aerobic fitness. However, it's all too easy to make a hash of planning a weekly training schedule and you may not realize your mistake until you are two weeks into your plan, when you discover you have bitten off more than you can chew. To avoid that, and to save you having to write your own plan, I have designed a twelve-week plan in this section for you to follow. All of the workouts and training methods involved are listed in the preceding chapters and use exercises detailed in the exercise library in Chapter 5.

Normally, when I write an exercise programme for one of my clients they are sat right in front of me so I can ask them about their exercise likes and dislikes, strengths and weaknesses, previous and current injuries, the amount of time they have to train and the equipment they have available. Obviously, in this book I cannot do this.

Subsequently, I have made certain assumptions while designing this programme. I have assumed that you have no current aches and pains, are moderately fit, have access to some rudimentary training equipment or are prepared to track down some of the cheaper options described in this book. I have also assumed that you, like the majority of exercisers, want to develop a higher level of all-round fitness and are able to commit to four or five workouts a week. Finally, I am making the assumption that, having read the chapters on the importance of warming up, cooling down and stretching properly, you will do these things even though I have not detailed them in the programme. Remember – if you don't have time to warm up you don't have time to work out!

If you find that any of the workouts listed are beyond your current level of fitness you should scale the workout down to suit your ability. If a workout calls for twenty repetitions of a given exercise but you can only perform ten in good form, err on the side of caution and don't overdo it. That extra bit of work may lead to an injury so make haste slowly.

For the cardio workouts I have denoted times rather than distances. This means that, whatever the workout, you can choose to cycle, run, row or swim as you see fit. Simply apply the cardiovascular training systems guidelines to whatever cardio activity you prefer to do. So long as you apply either heart rate or rating of perceived

Week/day	Monday	Tuesday	Wednesday	Thursday	Friday	Saturday	Sunday
1	Running burpee pyramid workout	Whole-body strength training	Fartlek 20 minutes	Rest day or stretching	Whole-body strength training	LSD cardio 24 minutes	Rest day or stretching
2	50/40/30/20/10 descending rep circuit	Whole-body strength training	Fartlek 22 minutes	Rest day or stretching	Whole-body strength training	LSD cardio 27 minutes	Rest day or stretching
3	Minute-drills	Whole-body strength training	Fartlek 24 minutes	Rest day or stretching	Whole-body strength training	LSD cardio 30 minutes	Rest day or stretching
4	Tabata interval circuit	Upper-body strength training	Tempo training 20 minutes	Lower-body strength training	Aerobic intervals 4 x 2 minutes/ 2-minute recovery	Upper-body strength training	Rest day or stretching
5	'Eat the biggest frog first' workout	Lower-body strength training	Tempo training 22 minutes	Upper-body strength training	Aerobic intervals 5 x 2.5 minutes/ 90-second recovery	Lower-body strength training	Rest day or stretching
6	Deck of cards workout one	Upper-body strength training	Tempo training 24 minutes	Lower-body strength training	Aerobic intervals 5 x 3 minute intervals/60-second recovery	Upper-body strength training	Rest day or stretching
7	Spartan circuit	Peripheral Heart Action circuit	Anaerobic intervals 6 x 30 seconds/60-second recovery	Rest day or stretching	Peripheral Heart Action circuit	LSD cardio 35 minutes	Rest day or stretching
8	Up and down again pyramid workout	Peripheral Heart Action circuit	Anaerobic intervals 8 x 35 seconds/ 45-second recovery	Rest day or stretching	Peripheral Heart Action circuit	LSD cardio 38 minutes	Rest day or stretching
9	Prisoner burpee ladder	Peripheral Heart Action circuit	Anaerobic intervals 10 x 40 seconds/30-second recovery	Rest day or stretching	Peripheral Heart Action circuit	LSD cardio 40 minutes	Rest day or stretching
10	Super-six circuit	Upper-body strength training	Fartlek 25 minutes	Lower-body strength training	Tempo training 26 minutes	Whole-body strength training	Rest day or stretching
11	Broken 100 m sprints plus ten-minute bodyweight challenge	Upper-body strength training	Fartlek 30 minutes	Lower-body strength training	Tempo training 28 minutes	Whole-body strength training	Rest day or stretching
12	Deck of cards workout two	Upper-body strength training	Fartlek 35 minutes	Lower-body strength training	Tempo training 30 minutes	Whole-body strength training	Rest day or stretching

No Gym? No problem!

exertion to your workouts you should be able to train similarly effectively whether you chose to pound the pavements or thrash your local swimming pool to foam!

If, during the duration of this workout, you are unlucky enough to become ill or pick up an injury (did you warm up properly?!) don't be a slave to the programme but, rather, take a few days off and let your body get back to normal. Once you feel like exercising again, have a few easy workouts and then slot yourself back into the programme, but go back a week or two. Building up gradually after a layoff will lessen your chances of re-injury and also minimize the return of post-exercise muscle soreness.

Record your workout performances in your training diary, details of which can be found on pages 195-6, as can a sample training sheet.

CHAPTER TEN

Nutrition for health and weight management

Nutrition is such a big and complex subject that really it warrants a book all to itself - that is if you want to delve into the chemistry of nutrition and how food affects your cells, organs and the systems of your body! However, it's more likely that you are more interested in eating to feel good, look good and function well and aren't actually that interested in the underlying nuts and bolts of nutrition.

In lots of ways, many of us treat nutrition like a television set or computer ... we don't really care how it works; we just want it to do the job we bought it to do, so in this chapter I'm going to lay out a basic guide to eating well but without delving too much into the underlying nutritional science. While I intend to keep this section 'tech-lite' I can assure you that all my recommendations are based on sound scientific principles as well as lots of experience, both as an athlete and as a personal trainer/coach.

Base your meals around protein

When it comes to fitness, health and building a lean physique, protein is king. Exercise is catabolic; that is to say, it causes the breakdown of muscle tissue. Protein, which is digested and then turned into building blocks called amino acids, provides the means to repair this damage and help you recover from arduous workouts. Training hard without consuming sufficient amounts of protein is like trying to run wearing lead boots - you'll make slow or even no progress.

Most weightlifters and bodybuilders know about the importance of protein, but many endurance and general exercisers, as well as the generally sedentary members of the public, fail to consume enough. This is mainly down to what is typically considered as and promoted to be a healthy diet - one which is based predominately on carbohydrate. Carbs are certainly not the evil that some food manufacturers and weight-loss gurus make them out to be, but they have been over-emphasized for decades at the expense of protein.

The word protein comes from the Greek *protos*, meaning first or primary. Without the luxury of microscopes, MRI scans, blood tests and other such medical technology, many centuries ago, the likes of Hippocrates (often described as the father of

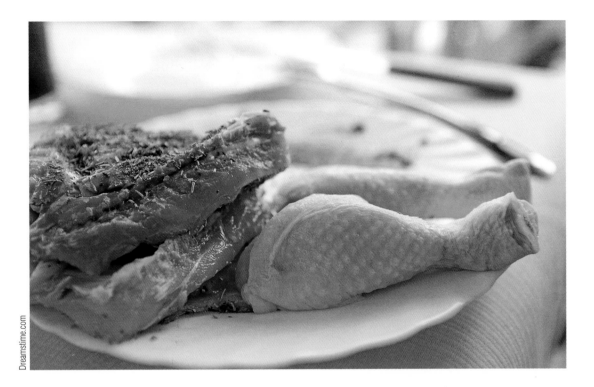

Dreamstime.com

medicine) figured out that protein was probably the most important food group for health and well-being.

So what foods contain protein? Good question! As a rule, if it swims, flies, crawls or walks (or could do when hatched in the case of eggs) it will contain protein. Dairy foods, being the product of said animals, like cows' or goats' milk, cheese and yogurt also contain protein, although unless they are 'on the turn' they should not fall into any of the preceding movement categories!

In addition to animal-based proteins, there are a number of meat-free protein-rich alternatives including beans, nuts, seeds and grains as well as soya and its derivatives.

When it comes to quality, not all protein foods are created equally. While the humble sausage may be mainly made from meat, the cuts of meat are not always the best. It's not that I have anything against sausages, pies, hamburgers etc., it's just that they tend not to contain as much protein as less-processed foods. The bottom line is that, like all foods, the less processed your protein is, the better it will be for you.

Protein can also be obtained by taking protein-based supplement shakes and bars. Just one word of caution: excess protein consumption – above the level that you need to support muscle growth and repair – can result in fat gain. Protein contains calories and while your body prefers not to convert unused protein into fat, if it is bombarded with too much protein for too long, that's exactly what it will do.

Animal foods, dairy products, some grains and nuts are good sources of protein

Protein supplements provide a convenient way to get protein into your diet but are not magical, nor are they essential. Most people should have no problem getting sufficient protein from 'real food'. If you do choose to use a protein supplement, remember, it should be considered supplemental to an already sound diet made up predominately of whole foods. It is not a shortcut around an otherwise poor diet.

So, how much protein do you need? The answer to that varies depending on who you speak to and what your ultimate training goals are. For sedentary people, it is suggested that they consume around 0.75 g per kilogram of bodyweight. For hard-working strength trainers, the most common recommendation is 2 g per kilogram of bodyweight. I believe that most regular exercisers should consume around 1.5–1.8 g of protein per kilogram of bodyweight (or a gram per pound if you are still working in imperial measures).

Carbohydrates – your energy supply for high-intensity exercise

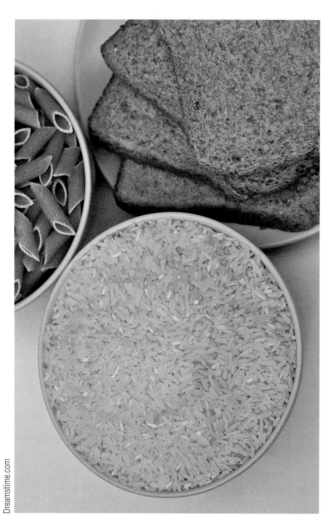

Dreamstime.com

Time your carbohydrate intake around exercise

The UK's National Food Guide and the Standard American Diet are very similar and suggest you should get the majority of your daily energy requirements from carbohydrates. Carbohydrate is an important fuel source for your muscles and your brain and the more active you are the more carbohydrate your body can effectively use. The trouble is, very few of us are active enough to justify eating a diet that contains sixty per cent or more carbohydrate (even if you exercise for an hour or so each and every day!).

Carbohydrate-based diets were actually a very good idea up until the time that the majority of the population stopped being so physically active. Carbohydrates – and this includes so-called low glycemic index or slow-releasing carbs – provide a fairly rapid source of energy. If you eat, for example, some bread, within a few short hours it will have been converted to glucose and be ready to be burnt as fuel by your muscles. The thing is, unless you are a building-site labourer or have a

No Gym? No problem!

similarly active job, that sudden influx of glucose is not going to be used. Long story short, unused glucose is converted very easily into fat.

If carbs are pretty much essential for fuelling your workouts but too much carbohydrate when you are sedentary can result in weight gain, what is the solution? I call it being carb smart. All this means is that you consume the majority of your carbohydrates before and after your workouts. The pre-exercise carbs will provide you with the necessary energy to train effectively while the post-training carbs will replenish lost muscle and liver glycogen (glycogen being stored glucose molecules bound to water). By doing this you ensure that you enjoy all the benefits of carbohydrate consumption without running the risk of weight gain during sedentary periods.

I'm sure you have heard of the terms simple and complex carbohydrates and refined and unrefined carbohydrates, but do you know what they mean? Allow me to explain...

In plain terms, **simple carbohydrates** are made up from one or two sugar molecules and include fruit, galactose (an element of dairy products), sucrose (table sugar) and other such things. Simple carbs can be healthy - as in fruit, or less healthy - as in confectionary bars, sweets and biscuits. All these things provide energy but only one provides vitamins, minerals and fibre in meaningful amounts and that's fruit.

Complex carbohydrates are made up of long, complex chains of glucose molecules and are often known as starches. Examples include grains like wheat and rice, vegetables and most other plant foods. As with the aforementioned simple carbs, complex carbs can be healthy or unhealthy. Wholemeal bread, for example, is considered healthier than regular white bread as it contains more fibre and is less processed.

The terms **refined** and **unrefined** simply refer to the degree of processing a food has been through. As a general rule, the more refined a food is, the less healthy it will be. I like to play this game when selecting carbohydrates and I call it the 'three steps to nutritional heaven' game...

When you look at a food, can you, in three 'moves', picture it or the majority of the food's ingredients in nature? For example, how many processing steps has your very convenient microwave meal been through? I'd guess at least a dozen! However, how many steps has wholegrain rice gone though from rice paddy to dinner plate? I think you get the idea! In general, you should try and eat foods that are as close to their natural state as possible. This preserves the vitamin, mineral and fibre content and ensures that the foods you eat provide not just energy but the biological spark-plugs that will keep you healthy.

When discussing carbohydrates, it's also important to know that carbs are your primary source of fibre. Without getting too heavily into intestinal health and the somewhat odious subject of faecal matter, fibre is essential for digestive health and is also a valuable weight controller, insulin regulator and all-round good guy. Most processed and refined foods are all but devoid of fibre and, while I don't suggest you become a 'fibroholic', I do suggest that you seek out high-fibre, unrefined foods to ensure you are getting enough of the good stuff. Leave the skin on your fruits and vegetables and select wholegrain (usually 'brown') grains and you should have no problem getting all the fibre you need to keep your digestive system in tip-top shape.

Don't be too fat-phobic

Fat often gets a bum rap in nutrition. If you take a look up and down your local grocery aisles you'll see countless low-fat products, which strongly suggests that fat is something that should be avoided at all costs. While it's true that fat contains a lot of calories (nine per gram as it happens, compared to four each for protein and carbs) and can make you fat, fat in itself is a lot less dangerous than we have been led to believe.

I'm sure you have heard the terms 'saturated' and 'unsaturated' fats/oils. These refer to how much hydrogen is in a fat and how stable it is. Saturated fats contain lots of hydrogen (they're saturated with it...) and subsequently they are very stable whereas unsaturated fats contain less hydrogen and are more reactive. Your body likes to use fat for energy and also as a source of stored energy but by and large fats are not as evil or as bad for us as we may have been told.

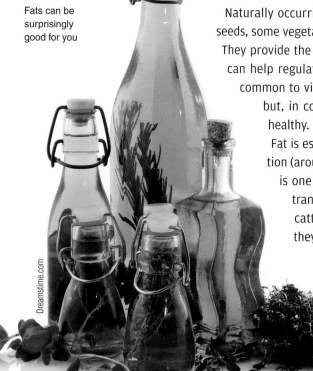

Fats can be surprisingly good for you

Dreamstime.com

Naturally occurring fats (obtained from animal products, nuts, seeds, some vegetables, etc.) are actually essential to your health. They provide the building materials for cells and hormones and can help regulate inflammation and blood glucose levels. It's common to vilify a diet containing moderate amounts of fat but, in contrast, a very low-fat diet is often much less healthy.

Fat is essential and can safely be consumed in moderation (around a gram per pound of bodyweight), but there is one form of fat that should be avoided and that's trans fat. In a western, trans fats would be notorious cattle rustlers wearing black hats. That is to say, they are the bad guys.

Small amounts of trans fat occur naturally and cause us no real problems but large amounts of trans fat can be very unhealthy and are linked to everything from obesity to cancer and from diabetes to heart disease. Trans fats are normally formed when unsaturated fats are processed (known as hydrogenation); this will turn a healthy natural fat into one that can do you harm.

The easiest way to ensure your trans fat intake is minimal is to a) use the 'three steps to nutritional heaven' process described earlier (page 163) and b) look out for terms like 'hydrogenated vegetable oil' in your food ingredients. Wherever possible, consume natural fats and minimize your intake of processed foods and you'll automatically decrease your trans fat consumption.

So, if fats (other than trans fats) are good for you, why all the hoo-ha linking them to poor health? Good question. In part, this is down to something called the lipid hypothesis, which is the result of research done by a scientist called Ancel Keys. Keys suggested that, after lots of testing, pretty much all fats were bad for you and should be consumed in small amounts only. In actuality, Keys based his studies on the consumption of too much trans fat - the real bad guy, as you now know. From his studies, he deduced that all fats acted the same way when consumed and tarred saturated, unsaturated and trans fats with the same brush when, really, only trans fats are proven to be harmful.

That's not to say you should go out and pick up a lard sandwich anytime soon! As mentioned, fat is very calorie dense and consuming too much fat can make you fat, which is very unhealthy. Rather than fear fat, choose unprocessed fats and eat them in moderation as part of your normal diet and only select low-fat options if you are concerned about overall calorie content. Cutting fat is an easy way to cut calories without reducing your food intake too drastically. I'll delve more into weight control shortly.

Eat the rainbow!

It seems that Mother Nature was labelling food long before food manufacturers started doing likewise. Instead of providing fat, calorie, ingredient and serving size information, Mrs Nature simply used colours to tell us what is in our food. In a nutshell, the more brightly coloured a food is, the more nutritionally dense it is likely to be. And, as different colours signify different nutrients, if you want to get a broad spectrum of vitamins, minerals and other healthy nutrients in your diet, you should try and eat a variety of food colours throughout the day - hence the title of this section. (Obviously I am talking about naturally occurring colours here! Don't for a moment think that just because you eat red, yellow, orange, blue and green jelly beans you are getting a healthy cross-section of vitamins and minerals!)

Personally, I like to see three or more different coloured plant foods in my main meals. I seek out reds, oranges, yellows, purples and greens and try to ensure that I mix and match over the course of a week so that I get plenty of what I need. The same colour advice can be used when selecting fruit - don't just go for the old standard of apples, bananas and oranges, try some less-common but brightly coloured fruits like fresh pineapple, cherries, pears, mangoes, star fruit or any of the other exotic fare now common in most high-street supermarkets.

As I have mentioned already, make a point of choosing food in as unprocessed a state as possible – that advice pertains to fruit as well. Fruit juices (made from concentrate, often with extra sugar and other additives) are not the healthy beverage you have been led to believe. In reality, many cartons of fruit juice are nothing more than liquid junk food and provide few, if any, nutritional benefits. If you do like fruit (or vegetable) juices and are consuming them for their proposed health benefits I strongly suggest you invest in a juicer and make your own. While the initial outlay may sting a bit, you'll then be able to make healthy juices using only the best ingredients rather than hoping that some faceless food manufacturer has left a modicum of vitamin C in your shop-bought juice carton. When it comes to juice, fresh is best!

Water – essential for life!

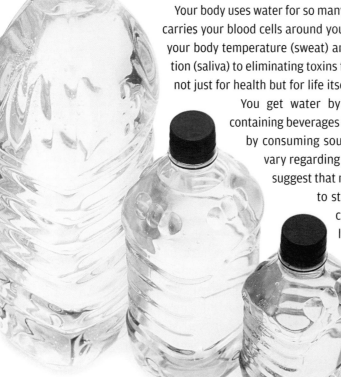

Dreamstime.com

Stay hydrated

Your body mass is made up of around seventy per cent water. While you can go for long periods of time without food, using your body fat for energy, you'll only last a couple of days at most without water. Of all the nutrient groups, water is the most important but often the least emphasized.

Your body uses water for so many things, from providing the medium that carries your blood cells around your body (plasma) to helping you regulate your body temperature (sweat) and from helping your taste buds to function (saliva) to eliminating toxins from your body (urine), water is essential not just for health but for life itself.

You get water by drinking water (!) and other water-containing beverages like juices, tea, coffee and soda, and also by consuming soup, fruit and vegetables. While opinions vary regarding how much water you need, most studies suggest that most of us need around two litres per day to stay healthy and hydrated. Of course, our caveman ancestors didn't know what a litre was (around 1.8 pints) and had to rely on their thirst to tell them when they needed to drink.

Luckily for our cave-dwelling forefathers, they didn't drink things like tea or cola, so their thirst was a much truer indication of hydration levels than our thirst tends to be. The thing is, we can

No Gym? No problem!

slake our thirst with non-hydrating fluids that do not actually increase our water intake. This means that, in modern times, prevention of dehydration through regular water consumption is the safest bet.

I have a small confession to make – I am a bit of a coffee addict. Not that freeze-dried stuff that comes in jars, mind you. Oh no, I only drink 'real' gourmet coffee made from freshly ground beans. Drinking coffee is pretty much my only vice and as I've gotten older popping out at night for a pint has been replaced by popping out at lunchtime for a coffee! I'm mentioning coffee for a very specific reason: because, although it is water-based, it doesn't contribute much to your actual water intake because caffeine has a marked diuretic effect, which simply means it makes you pee more than usual. This means that I don't count my coffee consumption when I am assessing my daily water intake. Nor do I count tea or the very occasional cola for the same reason and I suggest you do the same. Make sure you drink around two litres of good old plain water each and every day and consider other sources of fluid, like coffee and tea, as supplementary bonuses. That way, you'll be sure to be getting enough of what your body needs.

So, how do you know if you are dehydrated? If, other than your first urination of the day, your urine is dark and odious-smelling you are probably in need of water. If your lips are dry, your urine output is lower than normal, you have a headache or kidney-ache (often misdiagnosed as back-ache), these also suggest you are a bit dried out. If you are thirsty you may well be dehydrated but, as discussed earlier, thirst is a less then reliable indicator of hydration.

In addition to the standard two litres a day recommendation, I also suggest you drink 500 ml of water per thirty minutes of exercise to replace fluids lost through sweat and respiration. This means that, for many of you, you will actually end up consuming closer to three litres of water per day.

Of course, there is such a thing as too much water – something commonly referred to as water intoxication or, more properly, dilutional hyponatremia. This potentially fatal condition occurs when essential minerals become so severely diluted that your heart and brain cease to function properly. This is such a rare condition that it barely warrants discussion but, suffice to say, if you try and drink twenty-five litres of water a day you could very well make yourself ill.

No discussion on hydration would be complete without mentioning sports drinks. Sports drinks are often proclaimed as being all but essential and promise that they will allow you to train longer and harder than ever before. This is generally due to their carbohydrate content and is probably true if you are training for more than an hour or so. Most sports drinks also contain a group of minerals called electrolytes, which are commonly lost when you sweat. A drop in electrolytes can lead to muscle cramps and fatigue, but unless you are training in high temperatures, for extended periods, are poorly nourished or were dehydrated in the first place, it's unlikely your electrolyte levels should be major cause for concern. For the vast majority of general

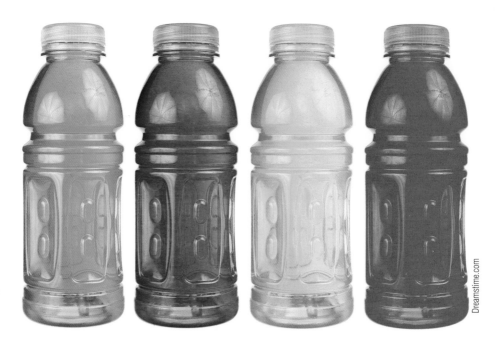

Sports drinks –
do you REALLY
need one?

exercisers, calorie-dense sports drinks are not only unnecessary but they provide an often unwanted source of energy that can interfere with fat burning.

If you are training normally and for an hour or less, water should be your beverage of choice during exercise. If, however, your training session is longer than an hour or you have been unable to consume adequate carbohydrate prior to exercise, a sports drink can be useful. Just don't be one of those overweight people I so frequently see plodding through their workouts while desperately sucking on a sugary sports drink - this is akin to eating while exercising and the chances are that they are putting in more calories than they are exerting. 'But it's a sports drink so it must be healthy!', they cry. Oh the irony!

Adjust eating frequency to suit your preferences

Ask a nutritional expert how many meals you should eat a day and you'll probably get the stock answer of three main meals and two or three light snacks. This means you will end up eating every two to three waking hours. In many ways, this is good advice. Frequent feedings have been shown to increase your metabolic rate, prevent hunger and keep your blood glucose levels on an even keel.

However, some research suggests that eating round the clock can down-regulate fat burning as your body knows there is a meal coming in the next hour or so, which means it has no reason to dip into its fat reserves. In addition, high-frequency meals may disrupt the normal hunger sensations.

As with all things nutritional, when it comes to meal frequency there is a broad spectrum of recommendations to consider. As mentioned, many experts stand by the six feedings a day protocol while others suggest that, as our cave-dwelling ancestors did, we would be better off eating one big meal at night and eating very lightly, if at all, during the rest of the day. Some go as far as to suggest that optimal health and longevity can be achieved by only eating every other day!

While I am not advocating fasting or even intermittent fasting I do think that many people eat out of habit rather than out of necessity. Habitual overeating combined with a sedentary lifestyle will result in an increase in fat storage and it's all too well known how being overly fat can adversely affect your health.

So, regarding meal frequency, don't be a slave to convention; consider moving away from the commonly prescribed high-frequency eating. If you wake up and you really aren't hungry then just grab some water and head off out the door. If you end up experiencing a mid-morning energy crash then maybe skipping meals is not for you, but if you feel okay then maybe you will be quite happy eating less often. The bottom line is that, if missing a meal or two was so bad for us, we'd never have evolved to where we are now as we'd all have died out from starvation. Many of the recommendations in nutrition are based on arbitrary numbers rather than iron-cast research so feel free to bend the rules, experiment and find out what works best for you.

Supplement wisely

Nutritional supplements are a controversial subject. Some people believe that you should supplement your diet with a myriad of vitamins, minerals and herbs to achieve optimal health while others suggest that, in actuality, you should get everything you need from 'real food' as Mother Nature intended.

While I think you should be able to cover the majority of your nutritional requirements within your normal diet, it's important to realize that food is not as nutritionally dense as it once was. Hundreds of years of intense farming and agricultural advances that allow crops to grow quicker and more frequently than ever before is resulting in reduced soil quality. Reduced soil quality results in less healthy plants and less healthy plants contain fewer essential nutrients. Because of regional variation it is impossible to say exactly how much less nutritionally dense food is compared to yesteryear, but some experts propose that modern fruit and vegetables are as much as fifty per cent less nutritionally dense. That's why, for many individuals, nutritional supplementation may be a good idea.

While I am semi-pro-nutritional supplements, I am less of a fan of so-called performance-enhancing sports supplements that promise bigger muscles, accelerated fat loss or increased exercise intensity. At best, these products are usually expensive and ineffective and at worse can be bad for your health. The main exceptions to this are a good-quality protein powder, as discussed in the protein section,

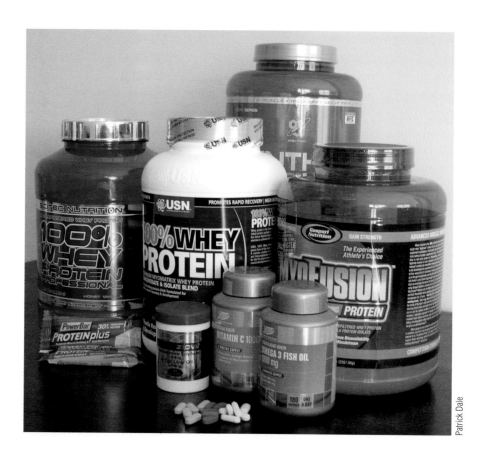

Supplements –
useful but seldom
essential

Patrick Dale

and creatine, which has been tested for over twenty years now and has shown itself to be effective.

While I'm on the subject of nutritional supplements, another thing I don't believe in is trying to prop up an otherwise bad diet with supplements. You can pop as many vitamins and minerals as you like, but you'll never out-supplement a bad diet. While nutritional supplements are often scientifically designed, they are no match for Mother Nature's nutritional masterpieces. If you want a complete and balanced intake of nutrients you need to eat a diet based mainly on whole foods and a variety of fruits, vegetables, whole grains, proteins and fats. Do that and you'll be ninety-nine per cent of the way there.

So, what supplements do I recommend? Firstly, recommend is a strong word and is very close to actually telling you to go out and buy a bunch of pills. I'm not prepared to do that (I'd need too much individual information to even begin such a process), so all I can tell you is the sorts of things I use and have used with my clients. Feel free to do some research and look up the various supplements discussed below to see if they would be useful to you, but also don't feel like you simply MUST take supplements. It's a personal choice and one you have to make for yourself.

No Gym? No problem!

- **Fish oil** - also known as essential fatty acids (EFAs), fish oils are rich in omega-3 fatty acids which are, unless you eat a lot of fish, commonly lacking in most people's diets. EFAs are linked to improved cardiovascular and brain health, lowered systemic and localized inflammation, improved insulin sensitivity, improved eyesight and better skin and hair. If I was only going to choose one supplement, I'd take fish oil. A good dose to shoot for is 1-2g. This should result in noticeable benefits in three to four weeks.

- **A good multi-vitamin and mineral** - a one-a-day multi-vitamin/mineral can provide a great nutritional safety net so, on the occasional day you don't eat as well as you know you should, you still have your nutritional bases more or less covered. Even the best multi-vitamin/mineral is only as good as its nutrient ratios and quality of its ingredients and none come close to 'real food', but if you feel like you need a nutritional security blanket, you could do worse than take one of these a day.

- **Vitamin C** - also known as L-ascorbic acid, this well-known water-soluble vitamin is strongly linked to immune system function and is also a powerful antioxidant. It can help minimize post-exercise muscle soreness and may even increase your resistance to certain viruses such as the common cold and flu. While the Recommended Daily Allowance (RDA) is only between 40-120 mg per day, there is significant evidence that suggests this range is far too low and, in actuality, 500-1,000 mg is required for optimal health. Either way, I know I get very few colds compared to non-vitamin C supplementing friends and I will continue to pop one gram a day for the foreseeable future.

- **Glucosamine and chondroitin** - being an older exerciser, I have a few aches and pains that are simply the result of over twenty-five years of vigorous activity. I've run miles wearing heavy boots and a rucksack, jumped on, off and over numerous obstacles and been on both the giving and receiving end of many a clattering football and rugby tackle. Subsequently, some of my joints are a bit on the creaky side.

     While creaks are okay, joint pain is not and so I, like many other joint-pain sufferers, take glucosamine and chondroitin. As well as being anti-inflammatory, there is some evidence that suggests that these two supplements (although they are commonly packaged together in one convenient tablet) may promote healing of articular cartridges. Either way, I know my knees feel less than optimal if I miss a few weeks of these supplements. Recommended dosages vary but I tend to favour the upper end of the scale and take between 1,000-1,500 mg a day.

Conclusion

The shelves at your local chemist or health-food shop are crammed with more supplements than you can shake a stick at so it's impossible for me to do justice to this enormous and, as I said, controversial subject in a few short paragraphs. If, having read this section, you believe you may benefit from some nutritional supplementation, do your research, make sure you buy the best-quality products you can afford, take them as directed and consistently monitor for benefits. If you don't feel you are getting much payback from your supplement use then maybe it's not one you need.

Fat loss and weight control

Whenever I open a magazine or newspaper I am astounded at just how much misinformation is printed about fat loss and weight control. Diet books are often a source of contradictory misinformation and the internet is literally drowning in fat-loss advice that is often ineffective, impractical and, in some instances, downright dangerous. Google 'fat loss' and you'll get in the region of 52,200,000 hits! It seems like good, honest fat-loss advice is becoming an endangered species and is being replaced by something far less useful – fad diets.

What is a fad diet?

Fad diets come in all shapes and sizes but usually share some common characteristics...

- They promise amazing fat-loss results in very short time frames
- They are endorsed by someone famous but not necessarily connected with the health and fitness industry
- They involve a very strict eating regime that is usually impractical and unappealing in the long run
- They require you to buy unusual or expensive foods and/or supplements
- They eliminate certain food groups while promoting others disproportionally
- They will leave you hungry, tired and feeling deprived of the foods you enjoy
- They are not designed for long-term use but, rather, to provide a 'quick fix'

The problem with any fad diet is that they only work because they are so restrictive. Unfortunately, the more restrictive the diet, the more likely you are to fall off the 'diet wagon' before you have reached your ultimate fat-loss goal.

In my time as a certified personal trainer, I have come to realize that the bigger or more dramatic the changes you make to your eating and exercise regimes, the more likely you are to revert to your previous unhealthy lifestyle. I call this the pendulum effect; the further the pendulum is swung away from the norm, the faster and harder it swings back again.

For example, you could embark on a fad diet that allows you to eat nothing but chicken and Brussels sprouts for the next six weeks. Every breakfast, lunch and dinner you sit down to a big plate of chicken and sprouts and nothing else. Initially, you will experience rapid and dramatic fat loss but, after a few days of eating such a restrictive diet, you'll get bored, feel deprived, become tired and irritable and most likely quit your diet and dive head first into a barrel of ice cream to cheer yourself up.

Using my pendulum theory, after such a big swing in one direction (the fad diet) you are much more likely to swing back to your old eating pattern and are going to end up eating even less healthily than before to make up for your period of deprivation.

When it comes to weight loss, if it sounds too good to be true, it probably is! Any diet that promises miraculously fast weight loss is going to have to be very strict and limiting, and while crash diets can work in the short term, for long-term health and leanness they are just about useless. In all my years in the fitness industry, I've only heard of a tiny handful of crash dieters boasting about their weight loss and how they then kept it off. The rest of the crash-diet gang tell horror stories of feeling weak, ill, lethargic and then, after all that sufferance, regaining the weight they lost seemingly overnight.

Why do crash diets fail to deliver meaningful and long-lasting weight loss? It's all down to something called the starvation response.

No need to starve yourself to lose weight...

When you go on a crash diet and dramatically reduce your calorific intake, your body or, more specifically, the hypothalamus region of your brain, doesn't know you are voluntarily eating less. It makes the assumption that food is dangerously scarce and takes steps to ensure you stay alive despite the lack of available nourishment.

Once this starvation response occurs, your body makes a number of changes designed to help you survive this period of calorific restriction. These changes include:

- Reducing your metabolic rate (the number of calories you burn per day) to ensure the little food you have goes further
- Using muscle mass for energy, which results in further lowering your metabolic rate
- Increasing the production of lipoprotein lipase – an enzyme that increases your ability to store fat
- Increasing your hunger levels to motivate you to get out and hunt (or hit the supermarket cookie shelves more like!)
- Reducing insulin sensitivity so that food consumed is more likely to be stored as fat

These mechanisms are designed to ensure your fat stores last longer, ensure that the little food you do eat is readily converted to fat and that you return to your previous level of fatness as quickly as possible. In many cases, crash dieters don't just regain the weight they lost, they gain back more as the body creates additional fat reserves to guard against future periods of starvation. This 'lose fat/gain more fat back' cycle is commonly called yo-yo dieting.

Sadly, there are no quick fixes to long-term weight loss. It takes most people years to gain excess body fat so it's going to take a while to lose it – especially if you want to keep it off. Most experts agree that, instead of trying to lose 20 lb virtually overnight, you should aim for 1–2 lb of weight loss per week. This is best achieved by making a small reduction in food intake and a small increase in activity levels. Such conservative interventions are sustainable for a long period of time and are very unlikely to trigger the starvation response. This way, when you reach your target weight, you won't experience a dramatic fat 'bounce back' and regain all the weight you have worked so hard to lose.

Rather than buying into the next celebrity-endorsed fad diet and setting yourself up for catastrophic failure, why not try a proven if less sexy option that is guaranteed to deliver results while allowing you to eat fairly normally? Moderation!

Moderation simply means eating a little better, eating a little less, exercising a little more and making these changes part of your everyday lifestyle for the rest of your life. Okay, so you won't lose 20 lb in two weeks, but the whole process will be much more enjoyable and you can still eat normal foods. You can even still enjoy treats from time to time – you just need to make sure that treats are an occasional rather than a frequent occurrence.

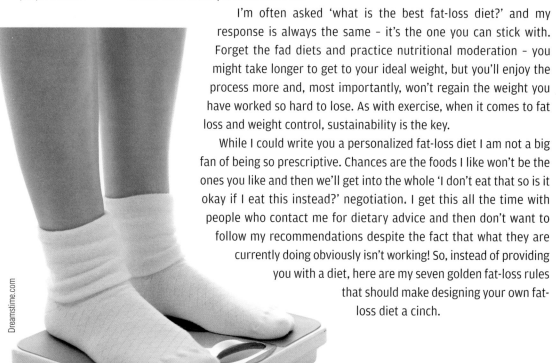

Weight control – one of the main reasons people exercise

Dreamstime.com

I'm often asked 'what is the best fat-loss diet?' and my response is always the same – it's the one you can stick with. Forget the fad diets and practice nutritional moderation – you might take longer to get to your ideal weight, but you'll enjoy the process more and, most importantly, won't regain the weight you have worked so hard to lose. As with exercise, when it comes to fat loss and weight control, sustainability is the key.

While I could write you a personalized fat-loss diet I am not a big fan of being so prescriptive. Chances are the foods I like won't be the ones you like and then we'll get into the whole 'I don't eat that so is it okay if I eat this instead?' negotiation. I get this all the time with people who contact me for dietary advice and then don't want to follow my recommendations despite the fact that what they are currently doing obviously isn't working! So, instead of providing you with a diet, here are my seven golden fat-loss rules that should make designing your own fat-loss diet a cinch.

No Gym? No problem!

One – eat protein at every meal

Take a look at most meals and you'll see they are built around starchy carbs like pasta, bread, rice or potatoes. There is nothing especially wrong with these foods but they aren't great if you want easy fat loss.

Protein, on the other hand, will really ramp up your metabolism, helps to preserve muscle mass when you are dieting and also keeps you feeling full for longer than carbs. By building your meals around protein you set your internal environment to 'fat burn' and away from 'fat storage', so make sure that the first thing you put on your plate is a good source of protein such as chicken, fish, lean meat, eggs or any vegetarian protein source such as quinoa, tofu or soya.

Two – earn your carbs

I discussed this earlier but it's worth repeating; carbohydrate is your muscles' preferred source of energy during exercise and, the more intensely you work out, the more carbs your body can use. Conversely, the more sedentary you are the less carbohydrate you need and any carbs consumed when you don't need them are easily converted to fat.

The best time to eat rice, bread, pasta and potatoes is one to two hours before and immediately after exercise. If you are taking a day off from exercise then cut down on your starchy-carb intake. On the days you work out include moderate amounts of starchy carbs in your pre- and post-exercise meals.

Eating carbs outside of this window of opportunity means that there is a fuel conflict and your body is more likely to use the carbs for energy, not your stored body fat. Limit your carb intake and you'll give your body no other choice than to burn fat for fuel.

Three – eat your veggies

If you follow tip number two, you need to make sure you follow this tip too! Cutting back on carbs is great, but you need to replace those carbs with something equally substantial if you are to avoid feeling hungry. Hunger can be abated by eating foods with bulk as they cause significant stomach distension, which makes you feel satiated.

Most veggies (with the main exception of potatoes) are very low in calories so you can eat a big pile of them without any worry of them interfering with your weight loss. Leafy green vegetables, mushrooms, courgettes, peppers, onions, cabbage, kale, carrots ... they're all filling and healthy and a major player in easy fat loss. Try to include a variety of colours in each meal so you get a broad spectrum of healthy nutrients. See how colourful you can make your plate!

Four – don't drink your calories

A typical can of regular soda contains around 40 g of sugar, which works out at around 160 calories. A blended iced coffee drink will contain even more sugar and a lot of fat too and can contain as many as 600 calories or more. Many fruit juice drinks are not much better...

The thing is, even the most calorie-dense drinks do not fill you up and often make you feel more hungry as they spike your blood glucose levels. This then results in a rapid increase in insulin production, which can ultimately leave you feeling deflated and craving more sugar. Save your calories for food and focus on drinking more water, unsweetened coffee and tea.

Five – be more active

So you have been following the workouts in this book – well done! You are doing more than the vast majority of the population and are well on your way to getting lean, fit and healthy. But; what about the 165 hours per week that remains? Do you spend the majority of your time sat down at work? Do you spend your leisure time sat watching TV or surfing the internet? Exercise is important for easy fat loss but most of us don't do enough general physical activity to be considered anything other than sedentary.

Your body is meant to be active for the majority of each and every day – something that very few of us are because of the passivity of modern living. For easy, starvation-free fat loss you need to seek out ways to be more active every day. Walk instead of drive, stand instead of sit, take the stairs and not the elevator, wash your car by hand, do some gardening, play with your kids ... do whatever you can to get up and get active. Adding this so-called non-exercise physical activity to your day will ensure that you experience faster, easier weight loss.

Six – minimize stress

Stress, be it emotional or physical, results in an increase in the production of the hormone cortisol. Cortisol can impair fat burning, increases insulin resistance (which limits your ability to use carbohydrates for fuel), promotes fat storage, reduces muscle mass and also suppresses anabolic hormone production. In addition, many people are 'stress eaters' and overindulge in less-healthy foods that will further compound the problems associated with elevated cortisol levels.

If you find it hard to lose weight or are showing signs of stress (inability to sleep, upset stomach, nervousness, anxiety, misplaced anger etc.) you should take steps to get a handle on your stressors and learn some effective coping skills. Exercise is a great stress-buster and so is mediation and deep breathing, but as stress is such a big and complex topic I can't do justice to it here. Luckily, there are lots of books and online resources that can tell you all about stress and how to deal with it.

Seven – treat but don't cheat!

One of the common features of very restrictive diets is the so-called cheat day. The basic premise is that you really toe the line all week, living on little more than a handful of mung beans and a few scraps of turkey, and then, to stop you losing the will to live, you are 'allowed' to pig out at the weekend. This 'strategic overeating', as it is euphemistically called, is often promoted as both a psychological and physiological benefit as it will rev up your metabolism and also give you something to look forward to each week.

While is true that your body will rev up to try and deal with the sudden influx of calories, it can only work on its highest 'setting' for a relatively short time. If the binge continues for too long, your metabolism simply slows back down to normal and body-fat levels start to increase again. It is not uncommon to hear of dieters who lose 5 lb in a week only to regain three over the weekend!

So, rather than being strict all week and going nuts at the weekend I suggest having smaller but more frequent treats if you feel deprived. This will hopefully avoid overindulgence and help keep your fat loss on the straight and narrow. So what constitutes a treat? Pretty much anything that does not fall into either the weight-loss or general-nutrition guidelines in this chapter. Cookies, cakes, crisps and chocolate are all good examples of treat foods.

Make sure you practice good portion control and, if you are anything like me, do not buy bargain packs of naughty foods with the intention of just having a little portion each day. Chances are, once you have had a taste you'll want more, so limiting the food you actually have in your cupboard will ensure you don't 'accidentally' go on a junk-food frenzy!

CHAPTER ELEVEN

Your common questions answered

I've tried to make this book as comprehensive as possible so that you can get in great shape without having to step into a big commercial gym or spend a fortune on fancy exercise equipment. However, the world of health and fitness is huge and is getting bigger every day. With this in mind, I have provided answers to some of the most common exercise, health and nutrition questions that I am asked in relation to exercising at home and fitness in general in the hope that I can address any concerns that may crop up as a result of reading this book. If you have any additional questions please email me at *patrickdale.militaryfitness@hotmail.com* and I will be more than happy to answer them for you.

A lot of the equipment you mention might well be okay for home exercise but if I buy it all it's going to be very expensive. Do I have to buy all that stuff just to get fit?
Absolutely not. You can develop a high level of fitness using nothing more than your body. I've included the exercises that use equipment, as I wanted to provide you with lots of options. If you want to train *au naturel* and use just your bodyweight then go for it – you'll get great results and save money as well.

How did you come to select the exercises and workouts detailed in this book?
All the exercises, and indeed the workouts, are the result of lots of trial and error. I have field tested all of the information outlined in this book. Exercises were selected on merit and the workouts listed are ones that I and my personal-training clients have enjoyed over the years. Equipment-wise, I have chosen training tools that are practical, versatile, effective, readily available and, wherever possible, cheap! I'm no armchair expert so don't worry – everything you read in this book has been successfully used by me and many other willing volunteers. It worked for us; it'll work for you!

Can I do your workouts at my gym? I like the ideas behind them but don't like training at home.
Many of the workouts listed can be performed in a gym if you so choose. In fact, despite having a good home-training set-up, sometimes I like to go to a gym simply

for variety. So long as you have space to exercise, ultimately it doesn't matter where you work out. One word of caution – some of the exercises will raise a few eyebrows as they are less than typical, so don't be surprised if someone comes and asks you about your new training regime!

I really want to make my muscles bigger and have heard that lots of cardio can interfere with this. What are your thoughts on this and what should I do to avoid this problem?

Too much cardio can certainly interfere with muscle building. I can attest to this personally. For years I struggled to gain muscle because I was a habitual runner as well as an avid weight-trainer. While in the Marines I suffered a stress fracture in my foot and so was unable to run for a few months. Needless to say, as soon as I nixed the running I found my muscle gain really took off. However, while I got relatively big and strong, I lacked cardiovascular fitness.

If muscle gain is your goal then have at it but include around three twenty-minute cardio workouts a week for the sake of your basic fitness and health. If, however, you want general fitness and strength, following the twelve-week plan outlined in this book will have you looking great and also developing a respectable level of fitness.

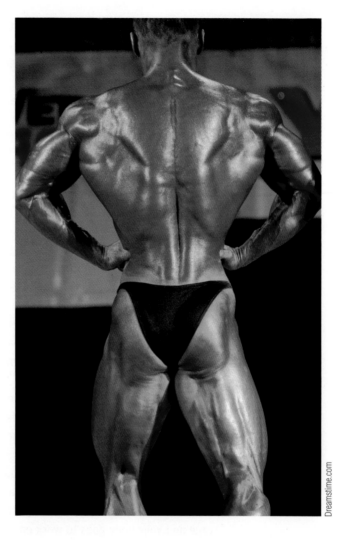

Dreamstime.com

Bodybuilding and lots of aerobic exercise often counteract each other

What if I can't perform the prescribed number of repetitions listed in the example workouts?

The repetitions listed are for illustrative purposes only so don't worry if you can't hit those numbers yet. Scale the workouts down to suit your current level of fitness. Maybe start by doing fifty per cent of the repetitions indicated and build up a little week by week until you hit the rep counts I have suggested. Focus on doing the exercises properly and with control; your fitness will soon increase and you may well surpass the listed rep counts.

I haven't exercised in years – can I still do your programme?

Yes – definitely, but do me and yourself a favour and get a check-up with your doctor first. I'm not trying to be a scaremonger; I just want you to make sure that you are healthy enough to exercise. Once you have got the all-clear then start exercising moderately but frequently. When you feel you have developed a base level of fitness you can start following the programme and workouts in this book. Remember, slow and steady wins the race so take your time building up both exercise intensity and volume.

I have a minor injury from working out – what should I do?

Firstly, if you feel anything untoward (that doesn't including sweating or panting!) you should stop what you are doing and call it a day. Pain means that something is wrong so you should never try to 'tough it out' or work through it. Next, get some ice on your injury. Always apply the ice to your limb – don't lay your limb on the ice – and use a medium, like a tea towel, between the ice and your skin to avoid the risk of ice burns. Apply the ice every three or so waking hours for fifteen to twenty minutes each time. After a day or so, see how your injury feels. If you are okay, start back with an easy workout and build back up over the coming week. If you are still feeing out of sorts then repeat the icing, rest a little longer and consider getting some medical advice.

Prevaricating slightly, if you are aren't injured but are feeling unwell then feel free to skip a workout or two until you feel a hundred per cent. Training while ill can make your illness last longer than it should do and will do little for your fitness.

I'm a terrible sleeper and only average around five hours per night. Will this hamper my progress and, if yes, what can I do about it?

Sleep is when your body goes through its recovery and repair processes. Hormones rage and your body goes to work ensuring you wake up fitter and stronger than when you went to bed, albeit very slightly. If you are not getting enough sleep you may well be compromising your fitness and even your health. If you have trouble sleeping it may be a good idea to speak to your doctor who may refer you to a specialist sleep clinic. Sleep-aid medication should be a last resort though as the side effects can outweigh the benefits. Make sure you are avoiding caffeine and excessive mental stimulation and try to set a sleep schedule to improve the quality and duration of your sleep. Finally, remember that an hour of sleep before midnight is worth two after – or so the saying goes!

Is this programme suitable for women and men?

Absolutely! I'm not a believer in training men and women very differently. In fact, one of the things that always gets my goat is seeing women who do nothing but group exercise classes and cardio and guys who do nothing but pump iron. Both

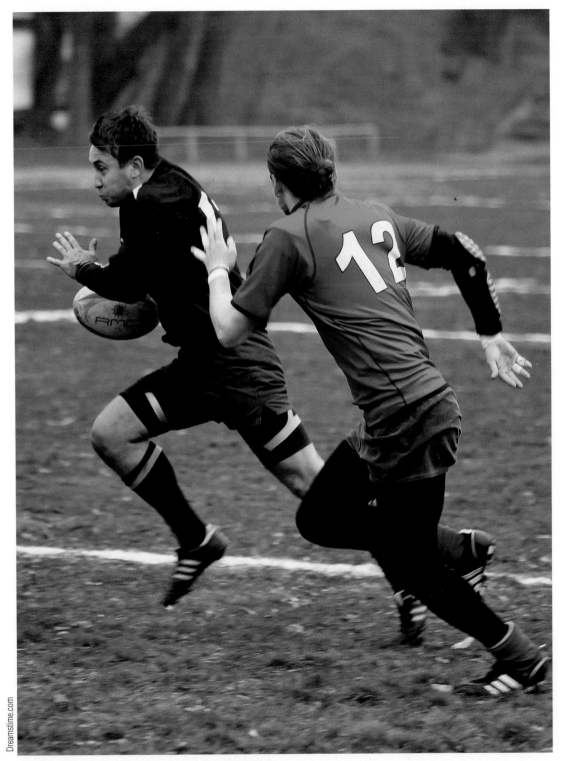

Whatever your sport, working out at home can and will work

sexes would benefit from crossing over into the opposite part of the gym – in most cases they'll reach their fitness goals much faster that way!

Women lack testosterone, the hormone that makes men manly, so don't worry about bulking up or gaining unsightly muscles. Building muscle is hard work and won't happen by accident.

My muscles are really sore after the first few workouts – am I doing anything wrong?

The only things you are probably doing wrong are exercising too much or too hard, too soon. Muscles soreness, often called Delayed Onset Muscle Soreness (DOMS), happens when you ask your body to do more than it is used to. While uncomfortable, it is not a serious condition, but you should really moderate your training to avoid excessive and unnecessary discomfort.

This also applies to returning to exercise after a two-week or more layoff. I've just got back from a holiday during which I did no exercise and, foolishly, jumped straight back into training at my normal level of intensity and duration. While the workouts were manageable, the post-exercise soreness I've experienced was spectacular! Don't make the same mistake I did – build up your workouts gradually over time.

Will this programme help me get fit for my sport?

Definitely! Although your sport probably has some unique demands, the generalized programme and training methods detailed in this book will help you increase your General Physical Preparedness (GPP), or all-round fitness, if you prefer.

What do you think of diets like the Zone, the Palaeolithic Diet, the Atkins' Diet and the Slow Carb Diet?

I often say that diet is a dirty four-lettered word as so many popular diets are unbalanced, overly restrictive and downright unpleasant. That being said, there are some good diets around if you want to learn about eating in a specific way or for specific goals like weight loss. Basically, a diet, no matter how many results it promises, will only work if you can stick to it. Not just for a day or a week, but for the foreseeable future. When considering any diet, ask yourself if you think you will be able to stick with it. If the answer is no, I suggest you look elsewhere. Also consider that many exclusion diets, i.e. those that 'ban' certain food groups, can end up being unbalanced and therefore potentially unhealthy as well as causing cravings for the disallowed food. That's why moderation is generally the best way to achieve meaningful and sustainable weight loss.

Isn't healthy eating more expensive than eating a 'normal' diet?

I don't believe it has to be but agree that sometimes it is. By seeking out low-cost but still healthy alternatives you should be able to construct a good diet for about the same cost. Admittedly, calorie-dense junk food is cheap, but then you get what you pay for - a whole lot of sugar and trans fat!

If you steer away from organic produce but instead just buy plenty of fresh fruit, vegetables, meat, fish and whole grains you should have no trouble eating well and staying within your budget.

Eggs – good or bad? And how many should you eat a day?

Not so long ago, lots of people were worried about the cholesterol in eggs and how it might be bad for your cardiovascular health. In part, this was due to the lipid hypothesis, which I told you about back in Chapter 10 (see page 165). The thing is, your body must have cholesterol to survive and your liver actually produces around 1,500 mg a day. If you eat eggs, and therefore ingest cholesterol, your body simply produces less to maintain balance.

Eggs are a cheap and convenient source of protein and essential fats, and are a good source of riboflavin, vitamin B12, phosphorus and selenium. As to how many eggs to eat a day, opinions vary but certainly a dozen a week should be fine unless you have some kind of underlying medical condition that means you produce more cholesterol than you should.

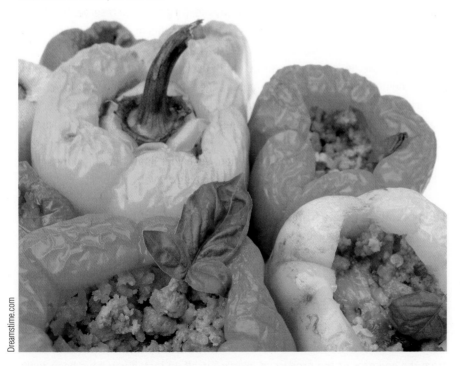

Dreamstime.com

Healthy food does not have to be boring!

Healthy eating? Dull! I'm sure that so long as I exercise I'll lose weight, get fit and look great on the beach! Or will I?

There is an old adage in exercise and nutrition – you can't outrun a bad diet. If you have got your calorie balance right and have built some muscle and dropped some fat, you will look good (hopefully), but on the inside, where it matters, your health may be at risk. Good health can be fleeting and is not something to be taken for granted. Just because one old chap lives to be a hundred despite smoking since the age of fourteen doesn't change the fact that millions of people die of smoking-related illnesses every year. Don't take the same risk with your diet. Eating a nutritionally poor diet can have a big impact on your long-term fitness and health and a bad diet will probably catch up with you in the end.

As for healthy eating being dull – it can be unless you make a point of learning how to cook and prepare tasty meals using good quality and healthy ingredients. It's not all salad and plain white fish, you know! There are plenty of healthy-eating cookbooks around so go and get one and learn how to make healthy food that tastes great.

How important is proper exercise form when working out?

I believe form is essential and insist on nothing but excellent exercise technique from my clients. Performing an exercise properly means you are less likely to suffer an unwanted injury and are also more likely to experience positive results from your hard work. Many trainers make a point of 'thrashing' their charges into a foaming and heaving mess, whereas I believe in always keeping a little in reserve. Tough, all-out exercise can be fun and exhilarating, but the benefits of doing that extra bit of exercise are more than outweighed by the risks.

For example, let's say you can deadlift 100 kg with good form. You attempt 110 kg and notice that your lifts are more ragged than normal and your lower back is starting to become rounded. The benefit of exposing your muscles to ten per cent more weight will be for nothing if you injure your back and are unable to train for four weeks!

Exercise conservatively and with caution. Push your limits but only nudge them a little at a time rather than kicking them up to a new level.

I don't really have any fitness goals except for staying fit. Am I doing myself an injustice by just working out rather than training for something more specific?

Training towards a specific goal can help keep you motivated and many people are very driven by the thought of setting new standards in their personal fitness. However, some people are process driven, which means they enjoy the doing rather than having a specific training target. So long as you gradually try to better yourself, week on week, year on year, it really doesn't matter whether your motivation comes from the end goal or the process of exercise itself. In fact, if you have been really working hard towards reaching a goal and feel like you need a break, it can be very refreshing to just train for fun, rather than pushing yourself day in and day out.

The bottom line is: choose whichever approach that floats your boat. If goal setting is not for you then no problem; so long as you are enjoying what you do then you will reap great rewards from your fitness endeavours.

Does this exercise lark ever get any easier? I've been working out for three months now and I'm still finding it hard!

I'm sorry to tell you that exercise never really gets any easier. The discomfort you feel as a beginner is pretty much the same discomfort felt by someone more advanced. The only real difference is the amount and intensity of the work performed. An unfit person's heart rate while jogging might be 150 bpm, the same rate as for an elite marathon runner running at top speed. Both will feel they are working hard (and both are, really) but the marathon runner is able to work at a higher level.

The same is true in strength training. Whereas a relatively weak beginner might be able to do ten press-ups but not eleven, a more advanced exerciser might do thirty but be unable to do thirty-one. Both will have worked as hard as they can to perform a maximum rep set of press-ups.

With the exception of DOMS, which tends to become less frequent and severe over time, exercise never becomes easy. But then it's worth remembering that nothing worth having comes easily – and fitness and health? They are definitely worth the effort.

When is the best time to exercise?

Some experts say that you should not lift weights first thing in the morning. Your body temperature is lower than normal, your blood glucose levels are down, your spine is not ready to support heavy loads and you are, in theory, more prone to injury. These same experts go on to suggest that that best time for strength training is mid- to late afternoon, so that your training session is preceded by at least a couple of meals, your blood glucose levels will be stable, your spine will be ready for action and you're likely to feel more 'up for it'.

Conversely, another group of experts suggest that, actually, exercising first thing in the morning is best. They say that as your blood glucose is low you are more likely to burn fat preferentially, that early morning training in a fasted state can boost your metabolism for the rest of the day and that you are less likely to skip a workout first thing in the morning, whereas exercising later in the day means that you might run out of time to work out.

So, as you can see, there is no unifying theory explaining the best time to exercise. I've done early-morning training, late-night training, midday training and even a mixture of all of these. As a triathlete I frequently trained two and even three times in a single twenty-four-hour period.

When it comes to the right time to exercise it really does come down to personal preference. Find the best time for you. This may take a little trial and error and you'll have to fit your preferred training time in with your daily schedule but, regardless, find a time and stick to it as much as you can. Make an exercise appointment with yourself and treat it as you would an appointment with someone else. While writing this book I made a point of stopping work at a specified time to exercise - even if I still had work to complete. It would have been all too easy to keep beavering away and end up running out of time and missing my workout. How hypocritical would that have been? By making a workout appointment you'll be much less likely to skip it.

How quickly can I expect to see improvements in my fitness?

Improvements in fitness can occur at different speeds. There are many factors that determine how long it will take for you to increase fitness:

- **Age** - the younger you are, the faster your fitness level is likely to rise. The unfortunate fact is that, as we age, our bodies take longer to repair themselves. This is compounded by changes in diet, changes in sleeping patterns and the natural hormonal decline associated with the aging process. When you exercise you are essentially breaking your body down. When you are at rest, your body builds and repairs itself, which translates into improved fitness and strength. In youth, these repair processes are carried out relatively quickly, but with more advanced age comes slower recovery. Also, as we age, our natural aerobic capacity goes down, as does the amount of muscle your body typically carries. The body simply becomes less efficient at physical activity. Don't let this deter you though - you can make considerable fitness gains whatever your age. Also, if you are over forty, consider picking up my book *Live Long; Live Strong* for lots of age-related exercise information.
- **Motivation** - I strongly believe that, the more motivated you are, the faster you will succeed. This is because you will notice even the smallest of improvements. A key to maintaining motivation is to set short-term goals that lead towards your longer-term goals. Short-term goals help you see the progress you are making. Keep a training diary and record your workouts so you can look back (with pride) at your progress. Nothing motivates like success and the more motivated you are the more likely you are to see significant improvements in your fitness.
- **Consistency** - this is arguably the most important factor in fitness. The best workout, the best diet, the most-advanced exercise programme are nothing but a lot of hot air if you don't have consistency. Long-term fitness and health are all about turning up day after day, and putting your time in at the coal-face of exercise. If you are consistent in your training, you will see your fitness improve before you know it. Results come after you dedicate

yourself to regular exercise. Don't take this the wrong way though - there is no reason to become obsessive. Obsession and dedication are not the same thing. Your fitness endeavours should enrich your lifestyle and not detract from it, as obsessive behaviour often can. Ultimately, consistency with a modicum of moderation will get you to where you want to be.

- **Rest** - there is such a thing as too much of a good thing. Chocolate, in moderation, can be healthy (if you buy the seventy per cent cocoa solids stuff!), but even something as packed with antioxidants as chocolate will do you no good if you eat a big family-sized bar every day.

  The same is true of exercise. While consistency is key, you also need to temper your efforts with adequate rest. Doing too much exercise can be as detrimental to your health as doing too little! If you do too much exercise and do not rest enough, you may end up suffering from something called overtraining syndrome, OS for short. Simply put, OS means that you are constantly tired, your immune system is compromised, your anabolic hormone levels are down and you start to feel less rather than more fit. As with many negative things, avoidance is your best option, so make sure your training week is peppered with regular days off. Even the most dyed in the wool exerciser doesn't need to work out more than five times a week.

- **Diet** - as you have read in the nutrition chapter, diet pretty much underpins everything that goes on in your body. You are, after all, what you eat. If you eat well and exercise sensibly you should see some significant improvements in your fitness and appearance quite soon after starting a new exercise routine. Conversely, if your dietary habits are less than optimal it stands to reason that your fitness may not improve as fast as you would like. I bet you wouldn't put dirty petrol in your car on purpose, so why do the same thing to your body? Eat well and your fitness levels will soon soar.

  So, how soon will you see improvements in your fitness? Pretty soon I'd say, but only if you get all your lifestyle ducks in a row and avoid the common exercise pitfalls. And even if your efforts only glean slow progress; so what!? Remember, you are doing this for you and you alone. Fitness does not need to be competitive.

What does the term 'empty calories' mean? How can a calorie be empty when it contains energy?

A calorie is a unit of measurement commonly associated with the amount of energy attributed to a specific food or foods. Obviously, all calories contain energy and so cannot truly be empty. However, the term empty calorie refers to foods that provide energy but do not bring anything else to the party; no amino acids, no fibre, no vitamins, no minerals. Like a freeloader at a 'bring your own bottle' party, empty calories use resources without providing any.

A good example of empty calories is refined white sugar. It contains plenty of energy in the form of carbohydrate (specifically sucrose), but is almost entirely devoid of nutrients. However, digesting and utilizing the energy in sugar requires vitamins and minerals so these have to be 'stolen' from your reserves. This is why empty calories are also commonly referred to as nutrient robbers.

Other common sources of empty calories include most sugary soft drinks, confectionary, refined baked goods, products made with refined white flour and any other foodstuff that has undergone aggressive processing.

While a calorie is never truly empty, those that are nutritionally poor should be made about as welcome as the bottle-less gate crasher!

I hate burpees – why are they so tough to do and why do you love them so much?!

How can anyone hate burpees? Or, rather, am I better off asking how anyone can love them? Love or loathe the burpee, there is no denying its ability to build fitness, burn calories and improve muscular endurance. I did 820 burpees in two hours to celebrate my fortieth birthday – that's how much I love them!

Seriously though, the burpee is so effective because it is so tough. Combining the squat, squat thrust, press-up and squat jump into a single flowing sequence means that you are using just about every muscle in your body, which places a tremendous workload on your heart and lungs.

I think my love of burpees came about when serving on board a navy ship as a Marine. The navy guys were generally not keen on fitness so the ships were often bereft of training equipment. With nothing more than a bit of space, I found that you can remain very fit (and lean) with little more than a liberal application of burpees.

Despite their lofty status as exercise royalty, burpees might not be for everyone. The deep squat, the dynamic leap out into the press-up position and a sky-high leap at the end means that for some, the burpee is simply an exercise too far. If this is the case, you can moderate the burpee by eliminating the press-up and jump and performing the exercise in slow time.

If you feel that burpees just aren't for you and you want an alternative, consider trying thrusters, high-pulls or kettlebell swings. These similarly global exercises work multiple muscle groups and will drive your heart rate sky high without having to perform a single burpee!

Your workouts are pretty unusual and not the normal thing I see people doing in the gym. Are your methods really that much more effective then more mainstream types of exercise?

Over the years I have been an endurance athlete, a long jumper and sprinter. I've climbed mountains, played rugby, fenced, competed in trampolining and diving and even scored over 220 while tenpin bowling! Because of these sporting experiences, I have been coached and trained by dozens of experts and each one has helped form my training philosophy. Combined with my experiences as a trainer, my studies and my time in the Marines, I have boiled down my theories on exercise into this unified no-frills approach to training.

Like Bruce Less says, 'Absorb what is useful and discard what is not', and that is what I have done. Everything in this book works and while I do not believe in cookie-cutter exercise programmes per se, I do believe that if you follow my guidance, you'll get more out of your workouts and save yourself a whole lot of wasted time and effort. Does that mean this book and my training philosophies will work for everyone? Absolutely not. But, within the confines of a book, it's impossible for me to provide customized workout solutions for all eventualities.

If you need additional guidance regarding any aspect of this or any of my other books, please contact me – I'm only too happy to help. Alternatively, you could pop over and visit me in Cyprus where I would be happy to train you personally!

I am about as flexible as a wooden plank but I hate stretching. I don't have any injuries so do I really need to stretch?
Let me tell you a secret; I hate stretching too. I find it dull, uncomfortable and really would rather just not bother. But then, when I do skip my stretching and I'm feeling pleased with myself for saving a few minutes a day, my body likes to remind me of why I need to stretch. In short, I start to feel rusty! Stretching helps keep your muscles and therefore your joints nice and mobile. The thing is, in your youth, that's how your joints *should* feel. However, as you get older, it soon becomes all too apparent that muscles and joints need regular tender loving care in the form of stretching.

There is no evidence that categorically proves that stretching will prevent you from suffering an acute injury, but I know from the clients I see that those with poor flexibility often find exercises requiring a large range of movement difficult and that a lack of flexibility can lead to chronic aches and pains.

To cure me of my stretching phobia I recently hired a yoga trainer to come to my house each week. Initially I was less than enthused, but after a few weeks of consistent practice I began to see (and feel) the benefits. It was like a bulb turning on in my head – the reason I didn't like stretching was that I never did enough of it to garner any benefits! Just dipping your toe into stretching by performing a few rudimentary toe touches will do nothing for your flexibility or your enthusiasm for stretching. If you are going to do it at all, you need to do it right.

So, to finally answer your question – yes, you really need to stretch, but you also need to do it properly and with a degree of commitment and consistency if you are going to get anything from it. Don't just go through the motions – stretch with purpose!

I like your book very much – have you written any others?

Thank you and yes, I have. My first book, *Military Fitness*, is all about developing a high level of all-round fitness so that you are 'fit for anything that life throws at you', as members of the armed forces generally are. It contains lots of information on training, diet and exercise equipment and a twelve-week plan designed to whip you into shape. My second book, titled *Live Long, Live Strong*, is a study of exercising and aging. Full of information about how diet and exercise can help hold back or even turn back the years, this is a great book for anyone serious about living a long, healthy and independent life.

Glossary

I hope I have managed to explain myself clearly but, in case I haven't, here is a list of many of the common exercise, health and nutritional terms that crop up frequently in this book. It's not exhaustive, but I think I've included all the heavy-hitters! If nothing else, you can have fun bamboozling your friends with your new vocabulary...

Adaptations – the changes your body goes through as a result of exercise

Aerobic exercise – exercise performed where fuel (specifically fat and carbohydrates) is used in the presence of oxygen. Long distance running, cycling and swimming are all examples of aerobic exercise

Agonist – the muscle responsible for a specific joint movement

Antagonist – the muscle that must relax to allow movement to occur. Also the target muscle in an exercise

Balance – your ability to keep your centre of mass over your base of support

Blood pressure – the amount of pressure exerted by your blood against the walls of your arteries. Measured in millimetres of mercury and assessed as a measure of health

BMI – short for Body Mass Index. A commonly used calculation that compares your height to your weight

Body composition – the relationship between your fat mass and your fat-free mass (bones, muscles and internal organs). Normally expressed as a body fat percentage

Burpee – the combination of a squat, squat thrust, press-up and leap into the air. A popular exercise with military and at-home exercisers

Calorie deficit – eating less food than you need to maintain your current weight. Creating a calorie deficit is viewed as essential for weight loss

Cardiorespiratory – pertaining to the heart (cardio) and respiratory system (lungs)

Cardiovascular – pertaining to the heart (cardio) and circulatory (vascular) system

Coordination – your ability to move your limbs smoothly and harmoniously

Core – the collective term commonly used to describe the muscles of the front, side and rear of the midsection

Creatine phosphate – also known as CP. This chemical, which is stored in your muscles, provides fuel for short, intense bursts of activity lasting around ten seconds. Taking the supplement creatine can help increase your stores of CP which may prolong activity slightly and may promote faster recovery from intense exercise

Dehydration – the condition of having too little water in your body, which can result in thirst, loss of performance, poor concentration and, in severe cases, unconsciousness and death

Diet – the sum total of everything you eat and also a restrictive eating pattern adopted for weight control

Endurance – the ability of a muscle or muscle group to continue working for extended periods of time without undue fatigue

Essential Fatty Acids – EFA for short, these are fats that are considered essential to health and are commonly obtained from fish oils and unrefined vegetable oils. Commonly taken in supplement form

Exercise variables – details that can be adjusted to increase or decrease overload, e.g. the amount of weight lifted, number of repetitions performed or time spent exercising

Fad diet – an unsustainable, quirky and often unpleasant eating regime normally associated with unsuccessful weight loss

Fartlek – Swedish for speed play, it refers to a mixed-pace aerobic workout

Flexibility – the range of movement of a joint as limited by the muscles that cross it

Heart rate reserve – a method for ascertaining training heart rate that takes into account your resting heart rate. Considered to be more accurate and personalized than the simple Karvonan calculation

Isometric – a muscular contraction where force is generated but no movement occurs and also a form of strength training

Intensity – the degree of difficulty of an exercise or training session. Too much or too little intensity can result in sub-optimal results

Interval training – periods of high-intensity exercise interspersed with brief rests

Karvonan theory – a simple calculation designed to ascertain your ideal heart rate during exercise

Kettlebells – spherical, handled weights that are round and can be lifted and swung in a variety of ways to increase strength, mobility and cardiovascular fitness

Lactic acid – the by-product of anaerobic exercise and thought to be the cause of burning muscles and fatigue when training at high intensities

Long, Slow Distance – LSD for short, this is easy-paced aerobic activity performed at around sixty per cent of maximum heart rate

Medicine ball – a heavy rubber or leather ball specifically designed for exercise

Mobility – the ease of movement of a joint or joints

Neutral – refers to running gait and means your feet roll normally

Overload – exposing your body to more exercise stress than it is used to so as to elicit a training response and therefore increase levels of fitness and/or strength

Participation Activity Readiness Questionnaire – PAR-Q for short, designed to assess your suitability to exercise. Should be completed before starting a new workout programme

Periodization – a long-term training plan that involves periods of hard exercise with periods of easier 'active recovery' workouts. Designed to ensure long-term progress is sustainable

Peripheral Heart Action – PHA for short, this is a circuit using a very prescriptive exercise order designed to increase cardiovascular fitness and muscle conditioning at the same time

Power – force generated during high speed

Pronation – refers to running or walking gait and means your feet roll inwards towards your big toe

Proprioception – your ability to know where your limbs are without being able to see them

Rating of Perceived Exertion Scale – RPE for short, these scales can be used to assess how hard an exerciser thinks they are working. The simplified scale runs from one to ten whereas the original Borg scale of RPE runs from six to twenty

SMART – a common acronym for Specific, Measurable, Achievable, Recorded and Time-bound, pertaining to goal setting

Specificity – when fitness adaptations occur according to the type of exercises performed

Stability ball – 45–85 cm-diameter inflatable balls used for core and other stability-developing exercises

Starvation response – a built-in mechanism designed to stop you starving when food is in short supply. Results in the lowering of your metabolism and increased propensity for weight gain. Commonly triggered by low-calorie or fad diets

Strength – the maximum force a muscle or muscles can generate

Sun salutation – a series of gentle exercises that flow into a sequence designed to warm up your body before exercise. Part of yoga practices

Supination – refers to running or walking gait, also known as under-pronation, and means your feet roll outwards towards your little toe

Supplement – normally refers to nutritional supplements, which are taken with a view to improving health. May also refer to a type of exercise performed specifically to add an extra dimension to a workout or address muscular balance

Suspension trainers – similar to gymnastic rings and used for bodyweight exercises. Ideal for home use

Synovial fluid – an oil-like substance that keeps your joints lubricated and also nourishes the articular hyaline cartilage

Tempo – also known as cadence, refers to the speed of movement when performing strength exercises. Raising a weight in two seconds and then lowering it in three would be expressed as a 2:3 tempo

Tabata training – interval training using twenty-second efforts and ten-second recoveries. A very intense form of interval training, which is often known as High Intensity Interval Training (HIIT)

Tempo training – also known as Fast Continuous Running (FCR) and Anaerobic Threshold training (AeT), tempo training involves maintaining your highest sustainable exercise pace while still remaining aerobic. Can also be considered 'race pace'

Time Under Tension – by calculating how long each repetition takes and multiplying that figure by the number of reps performed it is possible to calculate the exact length of a set, which is properly known as Time Under Tension or TUT

Training systems – a recognized set/rep/exercise scheme designed to make your workouts more demanding or more time efficient. Drop-sets, pyramids, super-sets and circuits are all examples of training systems

Volume – the amount of work (exercise) done in a specified time frame. Too much or too little volume can result in sub-optimal results

Sample food and training diaries

You can use a notebook, spreadsheet, app, online logbook or these pages to track your exercise endeavours and food intake. Record-keeping will make it much easier for you to track progress and stay focused. Make copies of these pages and store them in a folder or use them as templates for your notebook or spreadsheet. Whatever method of record-keeping you choose, the most important thing is that you refer back to your previous notes so you can keep an eye on your progress. As we used to say in the Marines, failing to plan means planning to fail', so put pen to paper or finger to keyboard and start recording your progress!

Using the training diary sheets

You can use these sheets to record information about all of the workouts contained within this programme.

- **Workout** – note the type of workout performed, e.g. cardio, circuit or strength training.
- **Exercises** – list the exercises performed.
- **Sets/reps** – record the number of repetitions and sets performed. Use short-hand if you like. For example, rather than writing that you performed five sets of twelve repetitions, use the notation 5 x 12.
- **Weight** – record the weights used so that you can keep track of progress. Use kilograms or pounds according to your personal preference. Tracking your weights means you'll be able to see your progress and you'll know what weights to use the next time you perform this particular workout. Not all workouts use weights so leave this box blank as necessary. I use the notation BW to indicate a bodyweight exercise.
- **Duration** – some workouts are against the clock so record the time it takes you to complete them here. You can also use this box to note the duration of your cardio sessions.
- **Recovery** – make a note of how long you rest between sets of strength-training exercises or laps of circuits. Try to reduce the length of your recoveries as you get fitter.
- **Observations** – record your general thoughts about how the workout went in this box. You might include information on the weather if you feel it contributed to your performance or make a note to remind yourself to use a heavier weight for next week's workout. If you had a less-than-optimal workout because you

	Workout	Exercises	Sets/reps	Weight	Duration	Recovery	Observations
Monday							
Tuesday							
Wednesday							
Thursday							
Friday							
Saturday							
Sunday							

No Gym? No problem!

made a mistake timing your pre-exercise meal, make a note of it here so you have no excuse for making the same error again.

Using the food diary sheets

There is no need to weigh and measure your food. Simply list the basic contents of each meal and approximate portion sizes. The aim of this exercise is not to record your calorific intake but to examine the types of food you are eating. In all actuality, if you eat the right *types* of food, the quantities become much less important. Make a note of your pre- and post-exercise meals and make use of the mood and energy indicators.

About the energy/mood indicators

Assess your energy and mood levels one hour after each meal by ticking the relevant symbol. If you are somewhere inbetween the specified levels, simply highlight the two symbols that best describe how you feel. For example, if, after breakfast you feel fairly energetic and in a good mood mark both ☺ and 😐. If you are feeling slightly below average but not rock-bottom, highlight 😐 and ☹.

☺ = Feeling very happy and/or energetic
😐 = Average feelings of happiness and/or energy
☹ = Feeling unhappy and/or lacking energy

If you are getting more ☹s and 😐s than ☺s then you may need to examine your diet and act accordingly. Midday and post-eating slumps in energy and mood suggest low blood glucose levels. Low blood glucose levels can be the result of consuming too little carbohydrate or a dip caused by the rebound effect of eating too much sugar. As a rule, stable blood glucose levels should score ☺ after ☺ after ☺!

	Meal one	Meal two	Meal three	Meal four	Meal five	Meal six
Monday						
Energy/mood	☺ ☺ ☹	☺ ☺ ☹	☺ ☺ ☹	☺ ☺ ☹	☺ ☺ ☹	☺ ☺ ☹
Tuesday						
Energy/mood	☺ ☺ ☹	☺ ☺ ☹	☺ ☺ ☹	☺ ☺ ☹	☺ ☺ ☹	☺ ☺ ☹
Wednesday						
Energy/mood	☺ ☺ ☹	☺ ☺ ☹	☺ ☺ ☹	☺ ☺ ☹	☺ ☺ ☹	☺ ☺ ☹
Thursday						
Energy/mood	☺ ☺ ☹	☺ ☺ ☹	☺ ☺ ☹	☺ ☺ ☹	☺ ☺ ☹	☺ ☺ ☹
Friday						
Energy/mood	☺ ☺ ☹	☺ ☺ ☹	☺ ☺ ☹	☺ ☺ ☹	☺ ☺ ☹	☺ ☺ ☹
Saturday						
Energy/mood	☺ ☺ ☹	☺ ☺ ☹	☺ ☺ ☹	☺ ☺ ☹	☺ ☺ ☹	☺ ☺ ☹
Sunday						
Energy/mood	☺ ☺ ☹	☺ ☺ ☹	☺ ☺ ☹	☺ ☺ ☹	☺ ☺ ☹	☺ ☺ ☹

No Gym? No problem!

Index

M

maximum heart rate test, 61
meal frequency, 168
medical questionnaire, 14
medicine balls, 52
  make your own, 52
monitoring exercise intensity, 57
mountain bikes, 69

N

nutrition, 160

O

overload principle, 16

P

periodization, 25
peripheral heart action training, 29
pre-exercise considerations, 13
programme templates, 139-43
protein, 160
pulse lowerer, 132
pulse raiser, 125
punch bags, 49
  make your own, 51
pyramids, 26

R

rating of perceived exertion, 57
recovery principle, 21
repetition ranges according to fitness
  goal, 139
resistance bands, 48
resistance training systems, 25-35
road bikes, 70
rowing machines, 73
running, 61
running shoes, 63

S

sample workouts, 144-56
sandbags, 36
skipping rope, 45
sledgehammer workouts, 40
specificity principle, 20
stability balls, 48
starvation response, 173
static stretches, 133-8
strength training variables, 18
sun salutations, 130, 131
super-slow training, 30
super-sets, 28
supplements, 169
suspension trainers, 38
swimming, 66
  equipment, 67

T

Tabata interval training, 81
talk test, 57
tempo training, 78
timed challenges, 35
total-body exercises, 114-23
training diary, 195
treadmills, 73
twelve-week workout plan, 157-9
tyres, 40

U

upper-body pulling exercises, 85, 98
upper-body pushing exercises, 84-91

W

warming up, 124
weight loss rules, 175-7
weighted vests, 44